Essential Obstetrics and Gyn
A GUIDE FOR POSTGRADUATES

T5-CVB-148

Essential Obstetrics and Gynaecology

A GUIDE FOR POSTGRADUATES

James Willocks

M.D., F.R.C.O.G., F.R.C.P. (Glasg).
Consultant Obstetrician and Gynaecologist to the Queen
Mother's Hospital and Western Infirmary, Glasgow.
Honorary Clinical Lecturer, University of Glasgow.
Examiner to the Universities of Glasgow and Edinburgh,
The Royal College of Physicians and Surgeons of Glasgow
and the Royal College of Obstetricians and Gynaecologists.

CHURCHILL LIVINGSTONE
EDINBURGH LONDON AND NEW YORK 1978

CHURCHILL LIVINGSTONE
Medical Division of Longman Group Limited

Distributed in the United States of America by
Longman Inc., 19 West 44th Street, New York,
N.Y. 10036 and by associated companies, branches
and representatives throughout the world.

First published 1978
ISBN 0 443 01390 X

British Library Cataloguing in Publication Data

Willocks, James
    Essential obstetrics and gynaecology.
    1. Gynecology 2. Obstetrics
    I. Title
    618   RG101   78–40111

Printed in Singapore by Huntsmen Offset Printing Pte Ltd

Preface

This book is designed as a practical aid to those preparing for the second part of the M.R.C.O.G. examination. This examination demands extensive reading and a wide clinical experience. It has been said that the candidates know more than the examiners and this is sometimes true, for they present themselves full of knowledge derived from recent reading of large textbooks and a wide variety of journals. What is demanded of a specialist, however, is that he should display not only knowledge but judgement. The profusion of medical literature can sometimes obscure clinical realities and it is as well to be reminded of these after the basic reading for the examination has been done. Many candidates fail not because of lack of knowledge of facts but because of a lack of discrimination in arranging them. It is always a mistake to omit to state simple and apparently obvious truths and a sense of proportion is required not only for examinations but for clinical practice.

Therefore, at the risk of seeming elementary, this book tries to present some basic clinical material in a concise and readable form. No attempt has been made to include everything. Some specialised subjects, such as congenital anomalies of the genital tract, have been left out entirely for excellent specialised texts are available. Perhaps the short essays presented here may induce the mood to reply to essay questions in the examination. The book might even be of use after the examination is over.

Contents

Part I Obstetrics

1

Antenatal care

PRINCIPLES AND PRACTICE OF ANTENATAL CARE

Antenatal care has two main objectives, medical and educational.

1. It is a form of preventive medicine. Regular attendance and treatment during pregnancy helps to maintain the woman's health, prevents anaemia, confirms normal progress, including normal fetal growth, facilitates the diagnosis of complications of pregnancy and prevents some of the difficulties of delivery, thus reducing maternal and fetal mortality and morbidity.
2. It is a form of health education. The doctor and midwife have a duty to allay the pregnant woman's fears, to instruct her in the care of her body, to inform her about the process of birth, the care of the newborn infant and eventually about methods of family planning. Repeated visits offer a unique opportunity for building up a personal relationship and feeling of confidence which are just as valuable as any technical expertise.

Selection of high risk patients
Now that the incidence of hospital confinement is so high, the traditional criteria for delivery in hospital are not so strictly applied. However, wrong selection of cases still occurs and may be associated with risks to mother and child. Not all hospitals have equal facilities: patients who require intensive antenatal supervision may need to attend a hospital which is equipped to offer this service and this may involve them in personal inconvenience. Particular thought should be given to the presence or absence of an adequate anaesthetic service and of a neonatal paediatric department in the place where babies at risk are to be delivered.

A particularly high risk group consists of women who are unwilling to take advantage of the services provided, who book late or not at all and who do not take advice. These are often either young, ignorant primigravidae or careless elderly multiparae from poor homes. Maternity departments need to devise a suitable form of outreach to contact these patients.

Women who require antenatal supervision and confinement in the best equipped hospitals include:

1. Age over 40.
2. Parity more than 5.
3. Bad obstetric history, of recurrent stillbirths, fetal abnormality or abortions.
4. History of repeated premature labour.
5. Major medical disorders such as cardiac disease, diabetes and severe hypertension.
6. Rhesus Iso-immunisation.
7. Intrauterine fetal growth retardation.
8. Multiple pregnancy.
9. Malpresentations.
10. Previous Caesarean section, myomectomy or hysterotomy.
11. Previous gynaecological operations such as repair of prolapse, stress incontinence, fistula or third degree tear.

Examination at the first antenatal visit
The woman should attend an experienced obstetrician as soon as possible after pregnancy is diagnosed. This is particularly important for the estimation of maturity (see below). At the first visit a careful medical and obstetric history should be obtained and a general medical examination should be made as well as a detailed obstetric examination. Blood and urine tests should be taken.

History
1. Previous serious illnesses, e.g. rheumatic fever, renal disease, tuberculosis.
2. Previous surgical operations – particularly abdominal operations.
3. Family history of multiple pregnancy, fetal abnormality, diabetes or hypertension.
4. Obstetric history, with details of date and place of birth, maturity of pregnancy, duration of labour, mode of delivery, birth weight and an account of any complications. Consultation of previous hospital records is often of great importance.
5. Menstrual history should pay particular attention to the date of the last period and the date of stopping the contraceptive pill.

General examination
1. Height, weight and general physical appearance.
2. Presence of oedema or varicose veins.
3. Condition of the breasts.
4. State of the teeth.
5. Pulse and blood pressure.
6. Heart sounds and murmurs.
7. Any evidence of respiratory disease.

Obstetric examination
This should be made with the woman lying comfortable and the bladder empty so that accurate abdominal findings can be recorded.

1. The height of the fundus uteri, if palpable, should be noted, as should the presence of any other abdominal mass.
2. The size of the uterus should be estimated on bimanual examination if the pregnancy is of less than 20 weeks duration. Any adnexal swelling should be noted.
3. Fetal parts may be felt by ballotement after 14 weeks.
4. The fetal heart can usually be detected by the ultrasonic 'doppler effect' using simple apparatus, from the 14th week.
5. The cervix can be inspected and a cervical smear can be taken, although opinions differ about the value of routine antenatal cytology.

Blood tests
These require 20–30 ml blood.

1. Haemoglobin.
2. ABO grouping.
3. Rhesus grouping and antibody titre.
4. Rare blood groups (e.g. Kell, Lewis).
5. Syphilitic serology (VDRL test).
6. Rubella antibody titre.
7. Serum alphafetoprotein (AFP) estimation if the pregnancy is between 15 and 20 weeks. If the first visit is at an earlier stage blood can be taken later at the correct time.
8. *Guthrie test* for phenylketonuria. A drop of blood placed on a specially prepared paper is later subjected to a *bacterial inhibition assay*.

Urine tests
In addition to simple tests, using reagent strips, for protein, sugar and acetone, a bacteriological examination should be made to

detect asymptomatic bacteruria. This can easily be done by the 'Dip-slide' technique, which allows the examination of large numbers of specimens, only the positive culture-medium slides requiring more detailed examination.

On conclusion of the examination, the obstetrician should outline to the patient the arrangement for further antenatal visits and indicate the facilities available to her. She is given a supply of iron and folic acid tablets (usually a combined tablet containing 150 mg iron and 300 μg folic acid) and may also be instructed to take fluoride tablets to aid the nutrition of her baby's teeth.

More detailed advice from a dietitian or a nursing sister specialising in breast feeding may be available. The patient is usually given some pamphlets on health during pregnancy.

The first antenatal visit is time-consuming for the patient and should not be overloaded with detail. More important, is to instil a feeling of confidence that she will be looked after with kindness and efficiency.

Examination at subsequent antenatal visits
These visits should take place at intervals of 4 weeks until the 28th week, then at intervals of 2 weeks until the 36th week, then weekly until delivery. Not all these visits need to be to a hospital antenatal clinic and it is common practice for alternate consultations to be undertaken by the general practitioner. If possible, the woman should come to hospital often enough to make her feel she is in familiar surroundings when the time of confinement comes.

At each visit to hospital the following observations should be made

1. *Weight in standard clothing.* The normal weight gain in pregnancy is 21 lb (9·5 kg). The gain in the first 20 weeks is 7 lb (3·2 kg). A further 7 lb (3·2 kg) is gained between 20 and 30 weeks and 7 lb (3·2 kg) is gained between 30 weeks and term.
   Excessive weight gain may indicate fluid retention and a failure to gain weight may indicate fetal growth retardation but so many exogenous factors (e.g. diet, vomiting, holidays) affect maternal weight that many are sceptical of its value.
2. *Haemoglobin.* It is most important to repeat the haemoglobin estimation at every visit. Fuller blood examinations can be made if low figures are obtained. By this means folic acid deficiency can be detected early. The need for parental iron therapy has been almost eliminated.

3. *Urine tests for protein and sugar (by reagent strips).* If protein is found a midstream specimen of urine is tested by boiling. If sugar is found on more than one occasion, a glucose tolerance test may be indicated.

4. *Oedema.* If present, the cause of the oedema should be elicited. Is it dependent oedema or generalised? Is it associated with varicose veins? Is it a sign of pre-eclampsia?

5. *Blood pressure.* Levels above 140/90 mmHg are usually considered abnormal. A significant rise above the blood pressure reading taken at the booking visit is particularly important.

6. *Abdominal examination* should include: estimation of the fundal height or, better, of fetal size in relation to gestational age; the presenting part and its level above the pelvic brim; any excess or deficiency in the amount of amniotic fluid; auscultation of the fetal heart.

7. In all cases the date of first fetal movement should be recorded.

8. All women with Rhesus negative blood should have tests for antibodies at the 28th and 36th week, or more frequently if indicated.

9. A pelvic assessment may be made at the 36th week although few would now use this to predict the method of delivery. In all cases of malpresentation or high presenting part it may be better to avoid pelvic examination until placenta praevia is excluded.

10. Sonar and X-ray examination may be used as indicated. There is much to be said for a programme of routine sonar screening to estimate maturity, locate the placenta etc., but facilities are not yet developed enough to allow this to be done on a large scale.

11. Antenatal care is largely a matter of routine but it should never become a mindless routine. Alert attention to detail and constant sensitivity to the feelings of the patient are essential throughout.

DIAGNOSIS OF PREGNANCY AND ESTIMATION OF FETAL MATURITY

Some of the clinical aspects of these subjects have already been touched on in the section on Principles and Practice of Antenatal Care but they are of such importance that they merit separate consideration. Practically every antenatal test which reflects the fetal condition is related to maturity and no intelligent use can be made of the tests if this basic fact is uncertain.

Diagnosis of early pregnancy

1. *Clinical*

The development of rapid, easy and almost universally available immunological tests has led to a neglect of the clinical features of early pregnancy which may lead to wrong diagnosis from time to time.

It is well to answer clinically two questions in every woman who attends:

    a. Is she pregnant?
    b. Is the pregnancy intrauterine or extrauterine?

The symptoms of early pregnancy (amenorrhoea, nausea, tingling of the breasts) are too well known to require detailed repetition. Often a woman may merely have a vague feeling of pregnancy which precedes other symptoms. Clinical signs include:

    a. *Breast changes.* Fullness and distension of superficial veins; darkening of areolae and turgidity of nipple; enlargement of sebaceous glands surrounding the nipple forming Montgomery's tubercles.

    b. *Bluish discoloration of vagina* due to venous engorgement is often present in the early weeks.

    c. *Pulsation in the vaginal fornices* due to the increased vascularity of the uterus.

    d. *Softening of the cervix* is present early but the excessive softness of the lower uterine segment is not marked until after the 6th week. Because of the softness of the lower uterine segment, it is difficult to follow the continuity of the cervix with the body of the uterus and thus they appear separate on bimanual examination (Hegar's sign). After the 10th week this sign gradually disappears.

    e. *Uterine enlargement.* The uterus becomes soft, cystic and globular and enlarges progressively. The fundus uteri is palpable abdominally at the 12th week. In patients previously delivered by Caesarean section, the uterus often seems to be at a higher level than in others. Any adnexal mass or tenderness should be noted on vaginal examination and may raise the suspicion of ectopic pregnancy.

    f. *Internal ballotement.* This sign consists of pushing the examining fingers sharply upwards in the anterior vaginal fornix – the fetus is pushed up towards the fundus uteri, but sinking again will be felt impinging on the fingers. The sign can be elicited from the 14th week.

g. *Fetal heart sounds* can be heard with the ordinary stethoscope from 20 weeks onwards. This is an absolute sign of pregnancy. The 'Doptone' or 'Sonicaid' ultrasonic fetal heart detectors, which utilise the Doppler effect are simple to use and give positive results from 14 weeks onwards.

2. Urine tests

The presence of Human Chorionic Gonadotrophin (HCG) in the urine of pregnant women has been used since 1927 as a means of detecting pregnancy.

Modern tests are immunological. Anti-HCG serum is prepared in animals: this serum is neutralised by the chorionic gonadotrophins in the patient's urine. The other reagent is a suspension of red cells or latex particles which are coated or primed with HCG. The latex slide test is very rapidly performed but the more popular technique now is the red cell test. This test ('Pregnosticon') depends on haemagglutination inhibition. It is performed as follows.

a. A fresh suspension of red cells primed with HCG is made up with the suspension fluid.
b. 0·1 ml of urine is added to an ampoule of anti-HCG serum.
c. 0·4 ml of the primed cell suspension is added to the urine/antiserum mixture.
d. The final mixture is shaken, then left to stand for 2 hours.
e. A clear brown ring indicates a positive result – this is because the primed red cells are not agglutinated by the anti-HCG serum which had already been neutralised by the HCG in the urine. The cells then settle in the test tube in the characteristic brown ring.

These urine tests are very sensitive. False positives may occur due to technical errors or in women over 40 years of age.

3. Sonar

Ultrasonography is the most accurate method available of diagnosing early pregnancy and gives more detailed information than any other. Reliable apparatus and a skilful and intelligent operator, are essential, however, if the technique is to realise its full potential.

a. A gestation sac shows up as a white ring within the uterus as early as 5½ weeks after the first day of the last period.

b. The fetus can be seen from 6 weeks onwards and its crown-rump length measured. The growth of the crown-rump length is very rapid between 6 and 14 weeks and predictions of maturity made then are therefore very accurate.

c. The action of the fetal heart can be shown on a time-position scan from 7 weeks onwards.

d. The placenta can be identified from 10 weeks onwards.

e. Absence of fetal echoes and fetal heart action on ultrasonography leads to the diagnosis of 'blighted ovum' which has been found to be much more common than previously thought.

f. Ultrasonic examination should be done in all cases where the uterine size differs from that expected from the dates.

Estimation of fetal maturity

If a woman attends during the first 12 weeks of pregnancy and has the clinical and ultrasonic examinations described, the maturity of the pregnancy can be assessed with accuracy. Unfortunately, only a small number of patients have these advantages.

Many difficult obstetric cases present for the first time late in pregnancy. The woman's recollection of her last period may be vague or even mendacious; she cannot remember when she first felt the baby move; the uterine size does not correspond with the alleged dates. In a case of this kind, antenatal monitoring tests will be valueless unless an attempt is made to assess maturity.

1. *Clinical estimation* of fetal size offers a rough guide at least to about 28 weeks but becomes increasingly inaccurate thereafter.

2. *Ultrasonic measurement* of the biparietal diameter gives a reasonable indication of fetal maturity up to 32 weeks but is not accurate in late pregnancy.

3. *X-ray.* The usual criteria for the radiological estimation of fetal maturity are

a. If the ossification centre at the lower end of the femur is present, the fetus is at least 36 weeks mature.

b. If, in addition to the femoral centre, the ossification centre at the upper end of the tibia is present the fetus is probably 38 weeks mature.

c. If the tibial centre is larger than the femoral the fetus is probably post-mature.

Remember that bony development may be delayed in the growth-retarded fetus and this may confuse the picture. A hyperflexed fetus whose skeletal maturity is less than expected from the dates is probably dysmature and may need to be delivered. Radiological maturity in all cases is only accurate within ± 2 weeks, i.e. within a month. This is not much better than clinical assessment.

4. *Amniocentesis.* Amniotic fluid tests are methods of estimating the functional maturity of fetal tissues and organs.

    a. *Maturity of fetal skin* can be assessed by staining the desquamated fetal skin cells found in amniotic fluid with Nile blue sulphate. If 10 per cent of cells stain orange the pregnancy has reached 38 weeks: if 50 per cent stain orange, the pregnancy is at term or beyond. Cornified cells predominate in amniotic fluid from 38 weeks onwards but it is difficult to say when they were shed.

    b. *Maturity of fetal kidneys* is reflected by increasing concentrations of creatinine and urea. If the creatinine concentration is 2 mg/100 ml the fetal kidneys are probably mature.

    c. *Maturity of fetal lungs* is related to the amount of fetal pulmonary surfactant (lecithin) in the amniotic fluid. Lecithin is difficult to estimate but the lecithin/sphingomyelin ratio (LSR) is easily measured by colour planimetry.

Respiratory distress syndrome is unlikely to occur in the infant if the amniotic LSR is 2 : 1 or more. LSR is widely used as a test of maturity before embarking on premature delivery but results should be intelligently interpreted; the amounts of both substances in the amniotic fluid may be related to volume and circulation of fluid and the site from which the sample was taken.

ANTENATAL FETAL MONITORING

Antenatal fetal monitoring is a fashionable concept but it is as well to ask who is to be monitored and for what. Clinical antenatal care is in itself a form of monitoring. Good antenatal care and selection of patients is the beginning of antenatal monitoring just as skilful clinical management in labour is its end. Funds available for health care are limited and at present there is neither enough staff nor equipment to offer all tests to all patients, nor would this be desirable.

Selection of patients for monitoring
1. Previous history of perinatal death.
2. Previous history of baby with mental or physical retardation.

3. Previous history of 'small for dates' baby.
4. Pre-eclampsia, hypertension or chronic renal disease in present pregnancy.
5. Diabetes.
6. Antepartum haemorrhage.
7. Multiple pregnancy.
8. Baby 'small for dates' clinically in present pregnancy.
9. Uncertain dates.

Objectives of antenatal fetal monitoring

1. If normal growth and development is present, to avoid unnecessary intervention.
2. To give warning of intrauterine risks to the fetus.
3. To assess the ability of the fetus to survive after birth.
4. To help in selecting the correct time and method of delivery, when it is apparent that the risk of continuing in utero exceeds the risk of extrauterine life.

Methods of monitoring

1. *Clinical*

Suspicion that antenatal progress and, in particular, fetal growth is not normal is an indication for starting tests. If the patient does not have one of the complications listed above under 1–7 the most likely reason for starting monitoring will be that the baby is 'small for dates'. When making this observation the obstetrician should note:

a. The fundal height, remembering that this is related to the level of the presenting part, e.g. if the fetal head is engaged in the pelvis the fundal height may seem low.
b. The size of the fetal head. Practice this method as a clinical gauge of fetal size.
c. The amount of liquor. If the uterus is tight around the baby, which is hyperflexed because of lack of amniotic fluid, dysmaturity is likely to be present.

If the obstetrician decides to admit the patient or submit her to further investigations, he should outline these clearly without causing alarm. If the investigations involve 24-hour collections of urine on an outpatient basis unequivocal and easily understood instructions should be given.

Despite the interest shown in fetal growth in recent years it is disturbing to note that quite a large number of small babies escape clinical detection.

2. X-ray

The role of radiography in antenatal fetal monitoring is confined to answering two questions.

a. Is the fetus skeletally normal? Always remember that failure of growth could be due to some congenital abnormality (e.g. achondroplasia).

b. Are there signs of fetal growth retardation? These are hyperflexion, oligohydramnios and perhaps retardation of bone age.

3. Sonar

Unlike the rather limited use of X-rays, ultrasonography with its safety, repeatability and increasing precision of anatomical definition offers boundless possibilities for direct communication with the fetus in utero. As has been shown, the diagnosis of pregnancy can be made ultrasonically within a few days of the first missed period and maturity can be established with certainty by measuring *crown-rump length* between 6 and 14 weeks. A prediction of maturity can also be made by a careful early ultrasonic measurement of the fetal *biparietal diameter*. Diagnostic ultrasound gives such valuable information about maturity that it is advisable to screen all patients with uncertain dates as early as possible in pregnancy.

Fetal growth in late pregnancy is best studied by *serial measurements of the biparietal diameter*. A fetus with a small biparietal diameter for gestational age, which on subsequent measurements is seen to be growing normally, may be a case of mistaken dates, whereas a fetus with a small biparietal diameter for gestational age which is not growing normally on repeated measurements is probably a true case of fetal growth retardation. Measurements are taken at weekly intervals: there is little point in making them more frequently as the growth over shorter periods is so small.

Biparietal cephalometry has become an established aid to obstetric practice in many centres. Other ultrasonic measurements of the fetus such as those of the thorax have also been used in combination with biparietal measurements to obtain a more accurate prediction of fetal weight.

Fetal breathing movements in utero have also been studied by ultrasound, both during pregnancy and in labour. A transducer strapped to the maternal abdomen directs a narrow ultrasonic beam towards the fetal heart, which is identified by its characteristic rhythm. Breathing movements have been reported as early as 13 weeks gestation. The number of breathing movements is said to be reduced in cases of diabetes and toxaemia and also during labour. A reduction in fetal breathing movements, or irregular gasping movements have been related to fetal distress as shown by late decelerations of the fetal heart rate and a fall in fetal scalp pH.

4. *Hormonal*

Hormones produced by the fetoplacental unit include oestrogens, progesterone, human chorionic gonadotrophin (HCG), human placental lactogen (HPL). There is a fairly wide normal range of all these substances during pregnancy.

a. Oestrogens. Oestriol is the most important in pregnancy. Its synthesis depends on both fetus and placenta. Most estimations of oestriol are based on an aliquot from a 24-hour collection of urine. Plasma oestriol estimations may eventually replace urine tests.

Oestriol levels are related to fetal weight and maturity, are low in pre-eclampsia, fetal growth retardation, fetal abnormalities such as anencephaly and are high in multiple pregnancy. Oestriols are of doubtful value in antepartum haemorrhage, diabetes and Rhesus iso-immunisation.

b. Progesterone. Urinary pregnanediol estimation was one of the first tests used for 'placental insufficiency', but has been replaced by oestriol estimations.

c. Human placental lactogen. HPL is produced by the placenta and is similar to pituitary growth hormone and prolactin. Plasma levels of HPL are measured by radioimmunoassay. HPL is roughly related to fetal weight, tends to be low in pre-eclampsia, high in diabetes and in severe cases of Rhesus iso-immunisation. It is said that some cases of intrapartum fetal distress and neonatal asphyxia can be predicted by low HPL levels.

d. Human Chorionic Gonadotrophin (HCG). Apart from its use in pregnancy tests there is little information on its value as a placental function test although it is produced entirely by the placenta.

5. *Enzyme analysis*

More than 85 enzymes are found in the placenta but only a few have any practical application and these are of limited usefulness.

a. Heat stable alkaline phosphatase (HSAP) comes from the cytotrophoblast. If results are abnormally low or rising rapidly in the third trimester, these may indicate danger to the fetus.

b. Diamine oxidase (DAO) in maternal serum increases rapidly to 20 weeks then more slowly to term. Its value is doubtful.

c. Cystine aminipeptidase (CAPO) is produced in the placenta and may be useful in predicting fetal death where pure placental dysfunction is the cause.

6. *Placental transfer tests*

The idea of measuring the transfer of a substance across the placenta as an indication of the function of that organ seems a good one, but the ideal substance has yet to be found.

Radioactive selenomethionine uptake is the only test which has been extensively explored. A low uptake ratio was associated with dysmaturity and fetal death. The test can only be repeated twice and there is uncertainty about its significance.

Placental uptake of technetium 99 is at present under investigation and it may help to identify growth-retarded babies.

7. *Stress tests*

Uterine activity and hypoxia can both affect the fetus in nature and to produce these effects in simulated conditions may be a valuable predictor of fetal behaviour.

8. *Fetal electro-encephalography*

Fetal electro-encephalography is at present a research technique but may develop into a useful method of preventing fetal brain damage.

FETAL ABNORMALITY AND ITS DETECTION

The great majority of severely abnormal embryos are discarded by spontaneous abortion. However, a substantial number of less severe abnormalities may survive. A congenital malformation may be defined as an anatomical abnormality present at birth and which may affect any organ or part of the body.

Congenital malformations have become relatively more important causes of death and disease among infants as other conditions have been successfully controlled. In 1900 congenital malformation accounted for 1 in 30 of infant deaths. At present they account for about 1 in 5.

The most important fetal abnormalities encountered by the obstetrician are:

1. *Down's syndrome (mongolism).* This is the only common malformation associated with a chromosomal abnormality, its usual form being Trisomy 21, i.e. these children have three No. 21 chromosomes and 47 chromosomes altogether. Occasional cases (about 2 per cent) result from translocation – an extra chromosome 21 being attached to another chromosome. Down's syndrome has an incidence of 1 in 600 live births and is responsible for about a quarter of all severely mentally handicapped children of school age. The newborn infant with Down's syndrome is characterised by slanting eyes with marked epicanthic folds confined to the inner angles: the bridge of the nose and the occiput tend to be flattened: the tongue protrudes: the hands are broad with short fingers and a single deep palmar crease: there is a large gap between the great toe and the second toe.

Young mothers rarely have babies with Down's syndrome but women over the age of 35 face a greatly increased risk.

In the maternal age group 35 to 39 years the risk of having an infant with Down's syndrome is more than 1 per cent while mothers over 40 face a risk approaching 5 per cent.

2. *Malformations of the central nervous system* cause the most deaths of all congenital anomalies, and surviving babies are usually severely handicapped, physically and mentally, despite recent advances in surgery. The commonest CNS malformations are:

a. Spina bifida with myelocele
b. Anencephaly
c. Hydrocephaly

The incidence of neural tube defects varies in different regions. It is high in Ireland and in the West of Scotland (6 per 1000 births). Anencephaly can often be suspected during pregnancy because of associated hydramnios and can usually be diagnosed by sonar or X-ray. Spina bifida and hydrocephalus were much more difficult to detect before the use of alpha-fetoprotein as a screening test. High levels of alpha-fetoprotein in the amniotic fluid in these cases are thought to be a direct result of leakage from the neural tube defect.

Risk of recurrence of congenital malformations – genetic counselling

Genetic counselling consists in giving as accurate information as possible on the transmission of inherited conditions and the risk of the birth of malformed infants or their recurrence.

Careful choice of words in communicating with the parents is of the utmost importance. There are very few cases in which the risk of recurrence is so great that they would be advised not to have a further pregnancy. Quoting recurrence rates in figures may not always be advisable as the risks of many conditions may not be great enough to prohibit further pregnancy or small enough to be reassuring. The effect of the advice given on the particular parents must be considered. Risks of the more important conditions are:

1. *Down's syndrome*
At maternal age 35–39 years the risk of mongolism is 1 per cent. Over the age of 40 the risk is 3·5 per cent. If both parents have normal chromosomes the risk of recurrence is equal to the incidence at the mother's age. The overall risk of *recurrence* of Down's syndrome is 0·7 per cent.

2. *Neural tube defects*
A woman who has had a previous child (or abortion) with spina bifida or anencephaly has a 5 per cent risk of recurrence. If two previous children were affected the risk is 15 per cent. If the woman herself has spina bifida the risk to her baby is about 3 per cent.

3. *Parental chromosomal translocation*
Most fetuses with unbalanced chromosomal translocations abort in the first trimester: the eventual risk of fetal abnormality is 13 per cent, rather than the predicted 50 per cent. Conceptions with a balanced translocation occur in about half the remaining pregnancies and, as the fetus is not severely handicapped, this is not an indication for termination of pregnancy.

4. *X-linked disease*
Where the mother is a carrier of an X-linked disease such as haemophilia or Duchenne muscular dystrophy, male fetuses have a 50 per cent chance of being carriers.

5. *Autosomal recessive metabolic diseases*
Although more than 60 inborn errors of metabolism can be detected antenatally these are very rare conditions. The chance of recurrence is 25 per cent.

6. *Cleft lip and/or palate*
A mother who has had one affected child has a recurrence risk of 4 per cent. After two affected children the risk is 12 per cent.

7. *Achondroplasia*

This is a single gene defect. Most achondroplastic infants are born to healthy parents and result from gene mutation. If one parent is affected by achondroplasia the risk to the offspring is 50 per cent.

8. *Cystic fibrosis*

Where both parents are carriers the risk to their child is 25 per cent.

External causes of congenital abnormalities (teratogenesis)

The literal meaning of teratogenesis is the causation of monstrosities. If the cause can be identified, prevention of further cases may be possible. The critical period for teratogenesis is between the 13th and 60th days of pregnancy – the period of organogenesis. Individual organs are susceptible at the time of maximum differentiation, e.g. at 4 weeks the limb buds are forming, at 6 weeks the palate is beginning to fuse and the primary fibres of the optic lens are laid down, at 8 weeks the septum of the heart is forming and the organ of Corti is undergoing spiral differentiation. Influences which may operate include:

1. *Metabolic factors*

Diet. There is no firm evidence that dietary factors are important. Vitamin A deficiency and Folic acid deficiency can cause congenital defects in laboratory animals but there is no evidence that humans are affected. A suggested link between potatoes and anencephaly has not been substantiated.

Diabetes. The incidence of congenital malformations in babies born to diabetic mothers is between 6 and 12 per cent. The cause of this is unknown. Insulin antagonists have been demonstrated more frequently in the mothers of infants with cleft lip and palate and spinal defects than in controls.

2. *Infections*

Rubella. The correlation between congenital cataract and maternal rubella was noted in 1941. In 1966, rubella virus was cultured from lenses removed from children of mothers who had had rubella. These observations show conclusively that a maternal virus can be transmitted to the fetus where it persists and can cause severe tissue damage. Other abnormalities induced by rubella include:

    a. Congenital heart lesions
    b. Deafness
    c. Mental deficiency

d. Thrombocytopenia

e. Hepatosplenomegaly

The total incidence of congenital malformations is about 20 per cent in those whose mothers have rubella in pregnancy. The virus does not appear to affect the fetus after the 16th week and after the 12th week the risk of malformations is slight.

As the clinical diagnosis of rubella is imprecise, if not impossible, it is advisable that pregnant women should have their blood screened for haemagglutination inhibition antibodies. If the initial titre is high and remains so 10 days later, immunity is presumed. If there is a significant rise in titre it may indicate recent infection. Complement fixation tests are confirmatory. Despite increased precision in the laboratory, great caution should be exercised in interpreting results as anomalous cases are not uncommon.

Women who are shown to be susceptible to rubella, but free from infection, should be immunised after delivery.

Herpes virus. Women may be affected by Type 1 herpes virus - in mouth, eyes or nervous system – or by Type 2 which is responsible for genital tract infections. In cases of genital herpes the fetus may be affected due to viraemia as well as by passage through the birth canal. Herpes may affect the child's brain, liver and adrenals but evidence of risk is lacking.

Influenza A. Inconclusive evidence of teratogenicity.

Mumps. Conflicting reports. Possible association with endocardial fibroelastosis.

Vaccinia can cause transplacental infection and fetal damage but this appears to be rare. Vaccination is best avoided in pregnancy.

Cytomegalovirus may be linked with microcephaly, chorioretinitis, deafness and mental retardation but more follow up studies are necessary.

Viral hepatitis. No teratogenic effect has been shown from either infectious or serum hepatitis.

Toxoplasmosis may damage fetal neural tissues but this is unproven.

3. Radiation

Ionising radiation is a very rare cause of congenital defect. Diagnostic doses of X-rays do not appear to be teratogenic although the link with childhood leukaemia is unresolved and every attempt should be made to avoid unnecessary radiation in pregnancy.

In the early days of medical radiology, when standards were less strict, microcephaly and mental retardation were reported as they also were in children who had been exposed to atomic bomb blast while in utero. Radioactive isotopes may be dangerous because they increase local tissue radiation to a very high level (e.g. iodine in thyroid, strontium in bones).

4. *Drugs*

One of the greatest risks of drugs in pregnancy is that women may take them at a time when they may not be aware that they are pregnant – and that is just the time when the risk of teratogenesis is greatest.

Two major types of toxic effect can be produced by drugs on the fetus – true teratogenic effects during the stage of organogenesis (e.g. thalidomide) or effects similar to those produced on adults (e.g. deafness due to streptomycin).

Most drugs cross the placenta; their transfer depends on the concentration gradient between fetal and maternal circulation, the area and thickness of the placental membranes, the rate of blood flow in the intervillous space and the molecular size and lipid solubility of the drug.

Many drugs have been shown to be harmful to the animal embryo. Few drugs have been proved to be teratogenic in humans.

The following drugs have been shown or suspected to be particularly dangerous in pregnancy.

Thalidomide. In 1961 reports from Germany and Australia showed a connection between previously rare major limb deformities (e.g. amelia, phocomelia) and maternal ingestion of thalidomide. About a quarter of the mothers who took thalidomide at the critical stage had deformed children. Some 4500 children in West Germany alone had thalidomide-induced deformities.

The teratogenic action of thalidomide was a surprise and is a warning against the reckless use of new drugs in pregnant women, for results of animal experiment may not be relevant to humans.

Progestational agents. These have been widely used for the treatment of recurrent abortion. It is doubtful whether they prevent abortion. It is beyond doubt that ethisterone and norethisterone can produce masculinisation of the female fetus – just like the effect of the related compound testosterone. There seems little justification for continuing progestational therapy for recurrent abortion.

The risk of contraceptive steroids giving rise to masculinisation of the fetus is so small that it can be ignored, but oestrogen/progestogen mixtures used as a means of diagnosing pregnancy can cause fetal abnormalities and these preparations should no longer be used.

Corticosteroids may be associated with a slight increase in the incidence of cleft palate. Cortisone and its derivatives should be prescribed in pregnancy only after careful thought. It is sometimes possible to stop long term steroid treatment (e.g. for skin diseases) during pregnancy.

Thyroid drugs. Treatment of the mother with antithyroid drugs and iodine-containing preparations may cause fetal goitre by blocking fetal thyroid hormone production with consequent over production of fetal Thyroid Stimulating Hormone (TSH). This effect is usually reversible. The effect of treating maternal thyroid disease with radioactive iodine (I^{131}) is irreversible: it is concentrated in the fetal thyroid and destroys it.

The diagnosis of hypothyroidism in the newborn must be made early if it is to be successfully treated.

Oral hypoglycaemic agents. Carbutamide and tolbutamide are teratogenic in rodents. No teratogenesis has been proved in humans but oral hypoglycaemics should be considered less safe than insulin for the pregnant women.

Anticoagulants. As oral anticoagulants cross the placenta there is a risk to the fetus – particularly from coumarin and indanedione derivatives. Parenteral heparin is the ideal anticoagulant in pregnancy because its large molecule does not cross the placenta, but its administration has considerable practical disadvantages.

Anaesthetics. There is no evidence to suggest that any of the commonly used anaesthetic agents are teratogenic when given in the course of a surgical operation. Investigations have suggested that chronic exposure to volatile anaesthetics may be a cause of an increased abortion rate among anaesthetists. Compounds chemically related to volatile anaesthetics are in use in industry (e.g. dry cleaning): so far there have been no reports of teratogenesis among workers.

Cytotoxic and immuno-suppressant drugs. These should not be used for the treatment of non-malignant conditions in pregnancy. Aminopterin and 6-mercapotopurine are teratogenic in animals. Cyclophosphamide, Chlorambucil and Methotrexate are also teratogenic in humans. Antimetabolites may cause fetal death.

Salicylates. Salicylates may precipitate neonatal kernicterus by displacing bilirubin from its combination with serum albumen.

Antibiotics. Tetracycline given late in pregnancy may discolour children's teeth. Sulphasoxazole has been suspected of producing embryopathy. No teratogenesis has been reported following the widespread use of antibiotics in early pregnancy (e.g. Ampicillin for urinary infection).

The detection of fetal abnormality

Antenatal diagnosis of fetal abnormalities may help towards a right decision regarding termination, may warn the obstetrician about complications of delivery and may facilitate early postnatal treatment. Congenital abnormality should be suspected clinically where there is:

1. A family history of congenital defects.
2. A previous abnormal baby.
3. A previous history of perinatal death or abortion.
4. Advanced maternal age and parity.
5. History of viral infections or exposure to teratogens in first trimester.
6. Diabetes.
7. An excess or deficiency or amniotic fluid.
8. Persistent fetal malpresentation or abnormal attitude, or failure to feel fetal head clearly.

In addition to clinical examination, the following antenatal diagnostic methods are available.

1. *X-ray* of the fetus helps to diagnose defects of the skeletal system – anencephaly, hydrocephaly, spina bifida and achondroplasia – but is sometimes not definitive, especially in the diagnosis of myelomeningocele, when the fetal spine sometimes looks normal.
2. *Sonar* can identify the fetal head at an early stage in pregnancy, certainly from the 12th week. Fetal heart action can be demonstrated from the 6th week. Anencephaly can be diagnosed with reasonable reliability and with the use of grey-scale techniques spinal defects are being identified.
3. *Fetoscopy*, the direct visualisation of the fetus by a fibre optic instrument passed through the uterine wall can demonstrate fetal anomalies but is a hazardous technique of limited application. Its chief use may be for sampling blood from fetal vessels to detect diseases such as thalassaemia.
4. *Amniocentesis* is the main diagnostic aid for the detection of fetal defects in early pregnancy and in experienced hands appears to carry little risk to mother or fetus. The main tests done are cytogenetics of cultured cells and estimation of alphafetoprotein (AFP) which reaches a peak at 16 weeks. Karyotype analysis takes about 18 days: the results of alphafetoprotein and sex chromatin determination can be available in 24 hours. The optimum conditions for amniocentesis are as follows:

a. Gestation should be 16 weeks. Earlier samples are smaller, more difficult to obtain, contain less viable cells and take longer to diagnose.

b. Amniocentesis should be done under sonar screening where possible. If amniocentesis follows ultrasonic localisation of the placenta immediately, samples (which should be 15–20 ml) are more easily obtained and less frequently contaminated with blood.

c. Samples, at room temperature, should be delivered to the laboratory as quickly as possible.

d. Kleihauer tests should be done before and after amniocentesis and all Rhesus Negative women without antibodies should be given 100 μg of anti-D gamma globulin after amniocentesis.

The risks of amniocentesis are:

a. Abortion. The abortion rate seems to be less than 2 per cent. Amniocentesis without prior placental localisation seems to be more dangerous.

b. Incorrect diagnosis. This may arise from growing maternal instead of fetal cells but is rare.

5. *Antenatal screening for spina bifida by maternal serum alphafetoprotein (AFP)* estimation has now been given an extensive trial following the development of radioimmunoassay technique. Grossly high values are found in cases of anencephaly and spina bifida but raised levels are also found in some cases of twins, threatened abortion and intrauterine death. A high rate of false negative results is found before 15 and after 20 weeks. The patient's gestation should be known accurately and should be as near 16 weeks as possible. Women who have had babies with previous neural tube defects, should be offered amniocentesis and amniotic AFP estimation irrespective of maternal serum AFP level.

If any patient has a raised serum AFP the test should be repeated before offering her amniocentesis. Only a raised amniotic AFP should be considered evidence of fetal abnormality.

Antenatal diagnosis of congenital defects allows abortion to be performed in cases where it seems likely that the child will be grossly abnormal.

The main hope for the prevention of congenital defects is in identifying environmental factors which may cause abnormal development.

2

Intrapartum care

NORMAL LABOUR

Stages of labour

Labour is traditionally divided into three stages.

The first stage. From the onset of regular and progressive uterine contractions until full dilatation of the cervix.

The second stage. From full dilatation of the cervix until the delivery of the baby.

The third stage. From the delivery of the baby to the expulsion of the placenta.

The uterus is active during all stages of labour, but, in addition to this, it is now recognised that uterine action in the later weeks of pregnancy is of great importance. This is the stage of 'Pre-Labour' or the 'Prodromal Phase' when the lower segment stretches, and the cervix becomes softer, is taken up and may begin to dilate. This process begins at about 30 weeks. The date of onset of spontaneous labour and the duration of the first stage are apparently related to the amount of softening and dilation of the cervix which is present before the onset of regular uterine contractions.

Onset of labour

The precise physiological cause of the onset of labour is not understood. A complex hormonal mechanism is obviously at work involving a reversal of the progestational phenomena which maintain the pregnancy and inhibit uterine activity. The process may be something like the following:

1. Fetal cortisol reduces placental progesterone production.
2. This enhances prostaglandin and oestrogen secretion.
3. The increase of oestrogen and decrease of progesterone enhance the output of oxytocin from the posterior pituitary.
4. Oxytocin acts on the myometrium and may increase the synthesis or release of prostaglandins.

5. Oxytocin inhibits the binding of calcium, thus increasing the amount of calcium available for combination with the contractile proteins of the myometrium. Contractions cannot occur without the presence of calcium.

Characteristics of normal uterine contractions
1. They are regular in rhythm.
2. Their strength and frequency increase steadily as labour progresses.
3. They have a 'plateau-like' form, pressure rising to a maximum, being maintained there for a period, then returning to the former base level. This means that the uterus relaxes completely to its normal resting tone, between contractions.

The pressures recorded during uterine contractions may be around 40–60 mmHg, whereas the resting tone of the uterus may be about 20 mmHg. A satisfactory rise of pressure during a contraction would thus exceed 20 mmHg. Recording of pressures gives only partial information on the work of the uterus. The function of the work done by the uterus is better expressed by the product of the amplitude and frequency of contractions, as in the Montevideo units.

Methods of recording uterine activity
Manual palpation
Despite the introduction of modern mechanical recording methods, the art of abdominal palpation during labour remains very important. Observations should be made for as long a period as possible by the same observer, although modern nursing organisation in the labour ward often militates against this. The frequency, duration and strength of the contractions should be recorded at 15 minute intervals and any change in their characteristics should be noted.

External tocography
Recordings of uterine activity made by devices strapped to the abdominal wall give information about the timing and, to a certain extent, the intensity of uterine contractions but do not record pressures within the uterus. External tocography has the advantage of being non-invasive.

The results depend on the thickness of the abdominal wall, the position of the recorder and also the position of the fetal parts and placenta.

Internal tocography

The advantage of internal recording of uterine activity during labour is that pressures can be measured. The method most frequently used is to pass a saline-filled fine open-ended plastic catheter inside the cervix at the time of rupture of the membranes. Blockage of the catheter is prevented by a slow flow of saline through it. A similar recording device can be passed through the abdominal wall, using a needle as for amniocentesis.

Numerous other intrauterine recording devices have been designed.

Methods of recording progress in labour

Clinical observations

Progress may be assessed by:

1. The increase in strength and frequency of uterine contractions.
2. The descent of the presenting part.
3. The dilatation of the cervix.

The dilatation of the cervix is the end result of all the powers of labour acting during the first stage and is therefore the most important single observation to be made in the assessment of progress in the first stage. It is not the only one worth making, however, and careful note must be made of the progressive nature of uterine contractions and of descent of the head otherwise serious clinical mistakes can occur – for example, an ill-judged attempt at vaginal delivery may be made as soon as the cervix is fully dilated, but with much of the fetal head still palpable above the pelvic brim.

Partogram

This is also a clinical method for it is merely a recording of the observer's assessment of cervical dilatation in centimetres set down on the Y-axis of a graph against time on the X-axis. Other features such as the level of the presenting part may also be recorded.

These recordings are highly subjective and depend on the experience of the observer. Unfortunately, the partogram is sometimes thought to have a scientific accuracy which it does not possess. It is, however, a useful way of depicting the pattern of the first stage and deviations from the normal pattern may be a guide in making the right clinical decision about the patient who is having a difficult labour. The partogram has been found particularly valuable in Africa, where mechanical forms of dystocia are common, for distinguishing patients who require intensive care in labour from those who can be classed as 'normal'.

Intrapartum fetal monitoring

The best way of monitoring the fetal condition in labour is by the complementary use of fetal heart rate recording (FHR) and fetal scalp blood sampling (FBS). These methods are best employed in obstetric units with more than 2000 deliveries a year so that staff gain sufficient experience in the techniques and their interpretation and that equipment is well maintained.

Fetal heart recording (FHR)

Combined systems for continuous recording of FHR and uterine contractions have come into common use in recent years. Various types of equipment are employed. A popular combination is that of direct fetal electro-cardiographic recording (FECG) using a scalp electrode with the use of an abdominal pressure transducer for recording uterine activity. Such systems have transformed the work of many obstetric departments and appear to have been associated with a reduction in perinatal mortality.

All fetuses are at risk and, where, possible, should be monitored in labour. It is not possible to select reliably a 'high risk' group and to relegate others to an inferior form of intrapartum care. It is essential that doctors and nurses who work in a labour room where fetal monitoring is practised should have the necessary skill in its management and in the interpretation of the results. Equipment for fetal monitoring should be safe and reliable and competent technical staff should be available to service it.

Methods of fetal heart recording. The fetal heart beat can be detected by the ordinary stethoscope, a microphone, an ultrasound beam or an ECG electrode system. The first is only applicable at intervals (usually every 15 minutes), the second requires the patient to be still and external noise to be excluded, so only the last two offer the opportunity for really continuous recording.

1. Ultrasound. Ultrasonic Doppler systems are directional and are therefore not particularly prone to interference from noise due to maternal movement: but fetal movement and a poorly defined time signal detract from the advantages of this technique.

2. ECG electrode system. The R wave from the fetal heart provides a very well-defined time marker lasting only a few seconds. This signal can be clearly detected by the application of an

electrode, usually a small stainless steel screw, to the fetal scalp. The time relationship between fetal heart changes and uterine contractions can then be studied.

Data obtained about fetal heart rate and uterine action are not completely understood, but there is general agreement that the following features are significant:

1. Slowing of FHR in relation to contractions. It is usually accepted that 'type one' decelerations, occurring at the same time as uterine contractions, are relatively harmless compared with the ominous 'type two' decelerations which occur a little later than the contraction which stimulated them, but it is dangerous to apply this as a universal rule.
2. A base-line FHR of less than 100 beats a minute, especially if it is falling, is a sign of fetal anoxia.
3. Loss of normal beat-to-beat variation in FHR is also considered a bad prognostic sign.

The significance of transient accelerations, decelerations and other changes in FHR is often uncertain. It is important to recognise that an abnormal FHR pattern is usually an indication for fetal scalp blood sampling.

Fetal scalp blood sampling (FBS)
There are biochemical changes in both fetal and maternal blood in labour. The most important measurement in both is the pH – which is practically the only measurement used in clinical practice.

In early labour, maternal hyperventilation causes a respiratory alkalosis which produces a rise in pH in the maternal blood. In the active phase of labour there is a metabolic acidosis which leads, by the time full dilatation is reached, to a pH value slightly lower than normal.

In the fetal blood, a pH of 7·25 is accepted as the lower limit of normal in the first stage of labour: during the second stage of labour a definite acidosis is usually present.

Experience has shown that it is reasonable to accept that the acid-base values of fetal scalp blood samples are a true reflection of the changes in the fetus.

Causes of fetal acidosis. There are two types of fetal acidosis, infusion acidosis and hypoxic acidosis.

1. Infusion acidosis occurs as a reflection of acidosis in the mother. This is an unusual cause of fetal acidosis in modern clinical practice.

2. Hypoxic acidosis. This is the result of fetal hypoxia for which there may be many causes including caval occlusion. Revealed caval occlusion manifests itself as the supine hypotensive syndrome, while concealed caval occlusion can occur in patients who maintain their systemic blood pressure by means of peripheral vasoconstriction. All patients in labour should be nursed on their sides or with at least a lateral tilt and it has been found that the fetal scalp pH will rise if the patient is turned from the supine to the lateral position.

Indications for fetal blood sampling
1. Anomalies in continuous FHR recording. For example 'type two' decelerations in FHR may be associated with a fall in pH to around 7·14. If the pH is normal and the FHR anomalies persist, the pH should be measured again in 30 minutes. If the pH is then still normal it can *probably* be accepted as more reliable than the FHR but it would be dangerous to ignore gross changes in FHR. There is little place for FBS in the second stage of labour: if the fetus is thought to be at risk then it should be delivered.
2. Meconium. FBS should be done if meconium is present. The chance of detecting meconium is an argument for early rupture of the membranes in all cases.

Technique of fetal scalp blood sampling
1. Place the patient in the lithotomy position with a 15° lateral tilt, or else in the lateral position.
2. Introduce the endoscope and press it against the fetal scalp, while an assistant steadies the fetal head by pressure on the maternal abdomen.
3. Dry the scalp with ethyl chloride spray and apply silicone grease.
4. Incise the scalp with the special knife so that a discrete drop of blood forms.
5. Collect samples in 2 heparinised capillary tubes.
6. Control bleeding from scalp by pressure.
7. Measure the pH of both samples on the Micro-Astrup.
8. Remember that results will improve with experience.

Intrapartum fetal monitoring should provide a rational basis for obstetric action and should sometimes provide reassurance so that unnecessary intervention is avoided. The interpretation of the data, however, remains difficult and is largely subjective.

Automated data analysis may help to produce more reliable information and it has been suggested that it might reduce the number of labour ward staff, but it is neither practical nor humane to leave labouring women without the attention of a nurse who, with proper training, can analyse the information provided by whatever monitoring system is in use and in addition can provide calm and comfort in a time of stress.

INDUCED AND AUGMENTED LABOUR

Induction of labour means the initiation of uterine activity by surgical means such as amniotomy, by drugs or by both methods. Augmentation of labour implies that once the uterus has started to contract spontaneously similar methods are used to speed the process.

Indications for induction

The classic maxim used to be that when the danger of continuing the pregnancy was greater to mother or child than the risk of induction, labour should be induced. Now that about 50 per cent of labours are induced in many maternity hospitals it is impossible to justify this approach in every case and there is no doubt that many women are induced around term with the object of securing increased convenience and efficiency for both patient and staff. The great increase in the practice of induction in recent years has been due to the development of more efficient methods. Recent publicity given to these methods has caused a certain amount of alarm and misunderstanding amongst women. It is the duty of the obstetrician to discuss frankly with his patient the arguments for and against induction in her case and to advise her with kindness and consideration for her feelings.

1. *Obstetric indications*
    a. *Pre-eclampsia.* There are risks to both mother and fetus and the timing of induction requires judgement, aided by knowledge about fetal maturity.
    b. *Eclampsia.* Labour should be induced once the fits are under control.
    c. *Abruptio placentae.* Particularly when the fetus is dead, induction is generally preferable to Caesarean section.
    d. *Placental insufficiency.* If evidence about poor intrauterine growth is certain and maturity is known. Some severe cases are best delivered by Caesarean section to avoid the hypoxic effect of uterine contractions.

e. *Rhesus iso-immunisation.* If the pregnancy has reached 34 weeks and delivery is indicated, induction, in spite of the risk of prematurity, is preferable to intrauterine transfusion which is reserved for less mature babies. Milder rhesus cases may be delivered at a later stage as indicated by spectrophotometry of the liquor.

f. *Fetal abnormality.* When gross abnormalities are diagnosed, pregnancy should be terminated.

g. *Intrauterine death* of the fetus is an indication for induction, which should preferably be medical to minimise the risk of infection.

h. *Hydramnios.* Induction may be necessary to give relief of pressure symptoms. The danger of abruptio placentae after amniotomy should be remembered.

i. *Postmaturity* has well known risks associated both with placental insufficiency and with dystocia. The main difficulty in these cases arises when there is uncertainty about maturity – for example, when the patient first presents late in pregnancy.

2. *General medical diseases*

a. *Chronic hypertension and renal disease* provide cases similar in nature to pre-eclampsia. Careful assessment and timing are essential.

b. *Diabetes mellitus.* Pregnancy is usually terminated about the 37th week, after which the risk of intrauterine death increases sharply.

3. *Epidemiological and social indications*

a. Women over the age of 30 years are said to face increased risks if their pregnancies go beyond term and it is increasingly common to offer them induction around their expected date. Certainly women over the age of 35 should not be allowed to go past term.

b. Poor social conditions. If women have difficulty in getting their other children cared for or if they live at a considerable distance from the maternity hospital, planned delivery on a certain date may be justified.

c. To ensure more efficiency and continuity of care it may be advantageous to offer the patient planned induction. The patient can then be attended in labour by the same team of medical staff who have been supervising her antenatal care.

Contra-indications to induction

1. A history of two or more previous Caesarean sections. Such patients are better delivered by repeat Caesarean section around 38 weeks to avoid the risks of ruptured uterus if labour starts spontaneously. Great care must be taken in the induction of patients with any previous operation on the uterus, e.g. Caesarean section, hysterotomy, myomectomy or any operations on the cervix.
2. Disproportion which is more than borderline. Such cases are now becoming more rare, but it would be foolish to induce labour in the presence of definite mechanical obstruction.
3. Where a tumour occupies the pelvis.
4. Where the lie is other than longitudinal or where there is a malpresentation such as a brow or face.
5. Cardiac disease is a traditional contra-indication to induction because of the risk of bacterial endocarditis but modern methods of intensive labour ward care have made this contra-indication less than absolute.
6. When the cervix is unripe, induction is less likely to be successful. If the indication for induction is a comparatively trivial one it may be postponed in the hope of securing more favourable conditions in a few days, but where serious obstetric or medical indications are present the plan for delivery should be continued despite the state of the cervix.

Methods of induction

The methods of induction in common use today are amniotomy, oxytocin and prostaglandins.

Amniotomy

Amniotomy has been used for more than 200 years and is remarkably effective even when used without any adjunct. Results from large series of cases show that about 80 per cent of women go into labour within 24 hours of amniotomy. Why rupturing the membranes should start labour is not clear. Changes in uterine sensitivity as well as volume are probably involved. The operation is a simple one when the fetal head is engaged and the cervix is ripe but it should not be performed in a casual manner or by inexperienced unsupervised staff.

The patient is prepared by having the bowel emptied by the use of suppositories and should arrive in the operating theatre with her stomach empty. Induction is usually performed in the morning and she should have no food from the previous night. This is an important precaution in case an emergency involving the use of general anaesthesia arises. Premedication with various sedatives and analgesics has often been recommended but this is unnecessary in most cases if the woman is treated with understanding, gentleness and skill. After confirmation of the lie and presentation by abdominal palpation and auscultation of the fetal heart, she is placed in the lithotomy position, the vulva is cleansed with an aqueous antiseptic solution such as 'Savlon' and sterile drapes are applied. The operator's hand is liberally smeared with antiseptic cream and two fingers are inserted into the vagina. The state of the cervix is assessed – its softness, degree of effacement and the dilatation of the os. The state of the cervix is probably the main factor governing success in the induction of labour. Where possible, a finger is inserted into the os and the membranes swept round before puncturing them with a suitable instrument such as the plastic 'Amnihook'. If the cervix is closed the membranes may be ruptured by the passage of a metal catheter: the old fashioned male metal catheter is probably less dangerous than the longer Drew-Smythe catheter. When the membranes are ruptured the colour and amount of the liquor is observed and a corkscrew type scalp electrode is applied to the baby's head so that continuous fetal heart monitoring can begin.

Risks of amniotomy include:

1. *Prolapse of cord.* This demands immediate Caesarean section. Fortunately, it is a rare complication (about 0·2 per cent).

2. *Supine hypotensive syndrome.* This may be associated with severe fetal bradycardia. Amniotomy should be performed as expeditiously as possible and the patient should not be left lying on her back too long. Supine hypotension can be corrected by altering her position.

3. *'Bloody tap.'* This may be due to placental damage (more common with the metal catheter) or to rupture of vasa praevia which can cause fetal exsanguination and death. If blood is obtained at amniotomy, a specimen should immediately be submitted for the alkali denaturation test which differentiates between adult and fetal haemoglobin. If the bleeding is of fetal origin, Caesarean section should be performed to save the baby's life.

4. *Amniotic fluid embolism.* The possibility of this rare but often fatal event should be borne in mind. The signs are dyspnoea, extreme collapse and massive pulmonary oedema.

5. *Infection.* Organisms from the bowel are present in the vagina of 40 per cent of women before induction and in a further 27 per cent after induction. The longer the membranes are ruptured the

greater the likelihood of intrauterine infection. This is one of the arguments for shortening the amniotomy–delivery interval by the use of oxytocin, but it seems from the results of large series of inductions that infection makes only a small contribution to the perinatal loss. Intrauterine infection is unlikely to be a problem if the induction–delivery interval is less than 18 hours.

Oxytocin
Oxytocin is generally used after amniotomy. The object in giving it is (a) to initiate effective contractions (b) to maintain normal pattern of uterine activity throughout labour. There are two main methods of giving oxytocin:

1. *The 'physiological' drip.* The theory on which this technique is based is that the concentration of oxygen in the blood necessary to initiate labour is the same as the concentration of anti-diuretic hormone required to inhibit water diuresis. In practice, a drip containing one unit of synthetic oxytocin to one litre of water is set up and the flow adjusted to 40 drops a minute (delivering 2·5 mu oxytocin a minute) and this rate is not exceeded. Advocates of this technique maintain that it is safe and that readiness of the uterus for labour cannot be provoked by massive doses of oxytocin. The disadvantage to the method is that the induction–delivery interval may be rather prolonged.

2. *'Oxytocin titration' or 'escalating oxytocin'.* This is the most popular present day method of giving oxytocin but it should only be used where facilities for fetal monitoring and tocography are available. Either a gravity-feed intravenous infusion or a motor-driven positive pressure infusion pump can be used.

The principle of the method is to start with a low dose of oxytocin, double it every 10 minutes until contractions begin, then double it again until regular, efficient uterine contractions are established. There is a wide range of response. An infusion rate of 10 mu/minute is often effective, but many patients may require 64 or 128 mu oxytocin per minute to produce adequate contractions. There is no doubt that this method shortens the induction–delivery interval but it is difficult to say whether it produces an increased Caesarean section rate. The rate of obstetric interference appears to be increasing and the unanswered question is whether this produces better results in the end for mother and baby. It is impossible to make a controlled scientific study because the more inductions are done the greater the proportion of favourable cases and the better the results. Oxytocin is a potent drug and high doses must be given with special care. Whatever method of giving oxytocin is used the drug should be continued throughout all stages of labour to minimise postpartum haemorrhage.

Prostaglandins
Prostaglandin was the name given to a substance extracted from seminal fluid which stimulated smooth muscle and lowered blood pressure. There are in fact a number of such substances. The prostaglandins which have been used in obstetrics are $PGF_2\alpha$ and PGE_2. The former was the first prostaglandin used in clinical practice but it produces unpleasant nausea, vomiting and diarrhoea and has been largely abandoned. Prostaglandin E_2 is a more effective preparation: there have now been a number of reports showing its ability to induce labour at term but it is not clear whether it is any safer or more efficient than oxytocin. Prostaglandin E_2 may be given by intravenous infusion, by continuous extra-amniotic infusion through a catheter passed into the cervix, or orally.

Like oxytocin, prostaglandins act best after rupture of the membranes but the extra-amniotic approach may be valuable when it is desirable to maintain the fetal membranes intact. PGE_2 may also be inserted vaginally in tylose gel. This has been shown to be a useful means of 'ripening' the cervix. The viscous gel acts as a slow-release vehicle. Oral PGE_2 appears to shorten the induction–delivery interval after amniotomy, particularly in the multiparous patient and may avoid the need for the patient having an intravenous drip.

The most favoured method of induction at present is amniotomy followed immediately by intravenous oxytocin usually given by the 'escalating' or 'titration' technique. Careful control of the drip rate is essential and this can be achieved by various automatic devices. Continuous fetal heart monitoring is also of prime importance if this method is used.

Augmented labour
The purpose of augmenting labour is to prevent prolonged labour and its dangers, which include infection, fetal asphyxia and maternal exhaustion.

The plan is to shorten spontaneous labour by rupturing the membranes and giving oxytocin. Proponents of this method maintain that it is safe, is associated with a low Caesarean section rate and avoids the need for large doses of analgesics.

The main cause of prolonged labour is *inefficient uterine action* and the remedy is to stimulate *efficient uterine action*. Classification of uterine activity as hypotonic or hypertonic now seems obsolete.

The possibility of cephalo-pelvic disproportion must be borne in mind but it should only be diagnosed once good uterine activity has been produced. Caesarean section has often been performed on the grounds of disproportion when the problem was really one of inefficient uterine action: this is particularly applicable to primigravidae. There can be no trial of labour without effective uterine action.

If a patient who is in spontaneous labour at more than 38 weeks gestation has poor uterine activity and the cervix is failing to dilate, forewater amniotomy should be performed and an oxytocin drip set up. These measures, together with effective relief of pain, will generally bring about a satisfactory delivery.

If oxytocin is used either to induce or augment labour it is important that there should be adequate nursing staff in the labour ward so that women are not left alone. Extreme caution is necessary if labour is augmented in highly parous patients.

RELIEF OF PAIN IN LABOUR

Most women require some method of pain relief in labour and some women later consider that the analgesia they had in labour was inadequate. The mental stress and tension which may accompany labour should never be underestimated. It is important to make a correct and safe choice of method in view of the needs of the patient and the facilities available.

Preparation for labour
There is no doubt that knowledge of the process of labour and confidence in the doctors and nurses who attend her is of great value to the woman in labour and reduces the need for drugs. Patients should know that efficient methods of pain relief are available and, in general terms, what these are. Complex psychoprophylactic and hypnotic methods may have their place but are not in general use. Any method which involves hyperventilation should be discouraged.

Sedatives and hypnotics
A sedative relieves anxiety and induces a feeling of calmness.

A hypnotic induces sleep resembling natural sleep. Patients in very early labour or on the night before induction of labour may benefit from a hypnotic. Barbiturates were widely used in the past but safer hypnotics are dichloral – phenazone (Welldorm) 2G or nitrazepam (Mogadon) 5 mg.

If the patient requires relief of anxiety in early labour, it is better to avoid oral drugs and to give sedatives by intramuscular injection. Phenothiazine derivatives such as promazine (Sparine) and promethazine (Phenergan) can be given in doses of 25 mg or 50 mg and diazepam (Valium) can be given in doses of 10 mg to 20 mg. It must be remembered that these sedative drugs have no analgesic action.

Analgesics

When uterine contractions become painful it is important that the first dose of an analgesic should be effective so that the woman's confidence is maintained. If the drug is given too little and too late, she becomes demoralised and analgesia is ineffective. Pethidine 150 mg is generally a suitable first choice and subsequent injections of 100 mg can be given. A combination of pethidine and a phenothiazine derivative may be indicated when anxiety is a prominent feature. When this combination is given, care must be taken not to produce hypotension, which is particularly liable to occur when the drugs are given intravenously.

Pentazocine (Fortral) 40 mg is an alternative to pethidine and is reported not to cause addiction. Both pethidine and pentazocine can produce respiratory depression in the neonate but this is seldom severe with normal dosage. Nalorphine and levallorphan do not reverse the effects of pentazocine. More depression is liable to be produced by morphine 15 mg but morphine still has a valuable place because of its powerful analgesic effect. Papaveretum (Omnopon) 20 mg is less liable to produce vomiting than morphine. Diamorphine (heroin) 5 mg may be used for an uncontrollable terrified patient. Narcotic analgesics and sedatives have no effect on uterine contractions and do not alter the progress of labour.

Narcotic antagonists

Narcotic antagonists are a necessary complement to the use of analgesic drugs as they can prevent or reverse neonatal respiratory depression. Levallorphan (Lorfan) and nalorphine (Lethidrone) have a chemical structure like morphine and compete successfully with the narcotics for receptor areas in the respiratory centre.

There is little justification for employing mixtures of analgesics and narcotic antagonists such as 'Pethilorfan' which had a transient vogue. It is better to administer the antagonist to the infant at birth.

Inhalational analgesia

Ever since Simpson administered chloroform in labour, inhalational analgesia has retained a place in obstetrics. The agents used nowadays are nitrous oxide, trichloroethylene (Trilene) and methoxyflurane (Penthrane).

1. Nitrous oxide is a powerful and safe analgesic if administered with enough oxygen. It is best given by the Entonox apparatus which has a single cylinder of premixed nitrous oxide and oxygen (50 per cent of each).
2. Trichloroethylene is a liquid anaesthetic chemically akin to chloroform. When given as an analgesic in labour by the Tecota or Emotril apparatus which deliver 0·35 per cent and 0·5 per cent of trichloroethylene vapour in air the effect is less rapid than that of nitrous oxide and the elimination of the drug is slower. Drowsiness and confusion are more liable to occur with trichloroethylene than with nitrous oxide.
3. Methoxyflurane is analgesic in similar concentrations to trichloroethylene – 0·35 per cent to 0·5 per cent and can be administered in the same way.

The advantage lies, in the writer's opinion, with the 50 per cent nitrous oxide oxygen mixture which is safe and should improve fetal oxygenation. The chief disadvantage of trichloroethylene and methoxyflurane is that they cause confusion and may make the patient difficult to control.

The place for inhalational analgesia is the late first stage and second stage of labour where, if efficiently given, it can be very effective.

Intravenous analgesia

When epidural analgesia is not available a continuous infusion of solution of pethidine (100 mg in 500 ml) will give more rapid and controllable analgesia than intramuscular injections. The pethidine in the drip may be supplemented by promazine, but the danger of this combination producing hypotension should be remembered.

Epidural analgesia

Where facilities are available, epidural analgesia is indicated whenever simple methods fail to relieve pain adequately. Its *advantages* are:

1. It usually gives *complete relief of pain.*
2. The patient is fully conscious and can take an interested part in her labour and delivery (spontaneous or operative) without fear.

3. The risk of aspirating stomach contents into the lungs, which is the most dreaded complication of general anaesthesia in obstetrics, is avoided.
4. Respiratory depression of the baby is avoided.
5. Epidural analgesia has a special therapeutic value in incoordinate uterine action, pre-eclampsia and heart disease.

The *disadvantages* of epidural analgesia are:

1. It requires skilled anaesthetic staff, available on a 24 hour basis, and patients need constant observation.
2. It may fail. This is usually for technical reasons. Dural puncture causes no serious harm if no injection is made.
3. It may produce hypotension: this can usually be avoided if the patient is nursed in the lateral position.
4. Rarely a high subarachnoid block may be produced, giving apnoea and profound hypotension. Immediate artificial ventilation is required.
5. There may be a toxic reaction to the local anaesthetic or an overdose which may be fatal.
6. There is a risk that signs of uterine rupture may be marked, especially in a patient previously delivered by Caesarean section.
7. It should not be given to any patient who is or could become hypovolaemic, such as a woman with antepartum haemorrhage, or to any patient with a bleeding tendency.

Technique of epidural analgesia
This is a difficult art. Epidural block should be performed only by one skilled in its use or acting directly under the supervision of an expert. This, in effect, mean that an efficient obstetric anaesthetic service should be available, not only because of the technical skill required in performing the block but because of the danger, remote though it may be, of complications. Only those able to manage an unconscious or apnoeic patient should conduct epidural analgesia.

At the start an intravenous infusion should be set up to allow for the rapid correction of hypotension. The patient sits on the edge of a tilting bed or table and is supported by an assistant who stands face to face with her. Identification of the epidural space depends on the fact that the pressure within it is subatmospheric and it is detected by the 'loss of resistance' technique – i.e. as the Tuohy needle, inserted into the interspinous ligament in the midline at L 2–3 or L 3–4, pierces the ligamentum flavum and enters the epidural space, there is a sudden sensation of 'give' and a small volume of solution can be injected with great ease. The syringe is detached and it is confirmed that neither cerebrospinal fluid nor blood emerges from the needle. The local anaesthetic is then injected: bupivacaine (Marcain) 8 ml of an 0·5 per cent solution is the most satisfactory. A plastic epidural catheter is threaded through and the needle is withdrawn. This allows for continuous epidural analgesia, subsequent 'top up' doses being given through the catheter in a sterile manner e.g., by using a sterile 50 ml syringe enclosed in a sterile plastic bag.

Management of labour with epidural analgesia
1. A high standard of nursing and great attention to detail is necessary.
2. The blood pressure should be taken every 15 minutes through-out labour and every 5 minutes for the 20 minutes after an injection. All attendants should know how to treat hypotension.
3. The patient should lie on her side whenever possible to avoid the supine hypotensive syndrome.
4. Intravenous fluids should be given.
5. Retention of urine should be looked for and treated as a full bladder may cause the patient no discomfort.
6. Uterine contractions should be monitored.
7. Oxytocin should be used when contractions are inadequate.
8. Regular vaginal examinations should be made to assess cervical dilatation. This is particularly important as the second stage approaches.

Other forms of regional analgesia

Caudal analgesia
The principle is the same as that of lumbar epidural analgesia but the injection is made through the sacral hiatus instead of the intervertebral space. This technique is very popular and successful in some hospitals but has been partly replaced in recent years by lumbar epidural analgesia which has a higher success rate, requires a smaller dose of local anaesthetic and involves entry through a less contaminated area of skin. The complications of caudal analgesia are the same as those of epidural analgesia.

Paracervical block
This means the injection of local anaesthetic into the areas of the uterine and pelvic (inferior hypogastric) plexuses of nerves at the sides of the cervix and body of the uterus. Because of the transient

nature of the analgesic effect (1–2 hours) and the problems connected with repeated injections, paracervical block is best administered late in the first stage of labour e.g. when the cervix is 6 cm dilated. In practice it can be difficult to choose the right moment for the injection. A needle with a blunt outer guide which restricts penetration to about 1 cm should be used. 10 ml of 0·25 per cent bupivacaine (Marcain) is injected transvaginally at the 3 o'clock and 9 o'clock positions in the vaginal fornices, after careful aspiration for blood. The main complication of paracervical block is fetal bradycardia and, rarely, fetal death has followed. This may be due to rapid absorption of the drug into the fetal myocardium but the mechanism is not entirely clear.

Paracervical block is a useful technique for the obstetrician who lacks the services of an anaesthetist and wishes to use regional analgesia for pain relief in the first stage of labour and for minor gynaecological operations.

Pudendal nerve block.
This method has been widely used for low forceps deliveries for about 20 years. The transvaginal approach is better than the transperineal. The ischial aspines are palpated and the local anaesthetic solution (e.g. 10 ml 1·0 per cent prilocaine (Citanest) is injected to a depth of 1 cm just behind each spine. Aspiration for blood should be done before the local anaesthetic solution is injected. The use of a blunt needle guide such as the 'Iowa trumpet' controls the depth of injection. Finally, the perineum is infiltrated along the line of the episiotomy.

Pudendal block does not always provide satisfactory analgesia for vaginal operations more complicated than simple low forceps deliveries. Other forms of analgesia, particularly epidural analgesia, are preferable for forceps deliveries involving rotation and for breech delivery.

General anaesthesia
General anaesthesia remains the most popular form of anaesthesia for Caesarean section but it carries considerable risk.

General anaesthesia accounts for about 8 per cent of maternal deaths in England and Wales. In Scotland, in the period 1965–71, general anaesthesia was associated with, although not necessarily the primary factor in, 12 per cent of maternal deaths. During the years 1972 to 1975, 7·6 per cent of maternal deaths in Scotland were due solely or principally to general anaesthesia. There were no deaths associated with any other form of anaesthesia.

The most important cause of maternal deaths under anaesthesia is aspiration of stomach contents into the lungs, because many such cases are avoidable. Mendelson's syndrome is an acute chemical pneumonitis due to the irritation of the lungs with acid gastric juice. Symptoms include severe pulmonary oedema and cardiac failure.

Prevention of deaths from pulmonary aspiration is by:

1. Diet. No solid food should be given to women in labour: if general anaesthesia seems a possibility no food or drink should be given. Many patients are on intravenous drips in any case and can receive adequate hydration in this way. A stomach tube cannot be guaranteed to empty the stomach: it is very unpleasant to the patient and it is better in general to avoid its use.
2. Alkali. Women in labour should be given 15 ml of magnesium trisilicate mixture every 2 hours and should have a further dose before any general anaesthetic. This should keep the pH of the gastric juice above 2·5, which is the critical level for the prevention of Mendelson's syndrome.
3. Regional or local analgesia should be used wherever possible.
4. Skilled anaesthetists should be available in all maternity hospitals.

The best technique of general anaesthesia for obstetric operations
The patient is on a tilting bed or table. An intravenous infusion is set up and 2 units of cross-matched blood should be available. Atrophine 0·6 mg is given intravenously as premedication. Pre-oxygenation is performed by the patient breathing oxygen through a mask for 3 minutes at 8 litres a minute.

Anaesthesia is induced with 150–250 mg thiopentone (Pentothal) followed by 100 mg suxamethonium (Scoline). Cricoid pressure is performed by an assistant to compress the oesophagus and prevent regurgitation. The trachea is intubated with a cuffed tube and anaesthesia is maintained with nitrous oxide and oxygen.

This is the safest technique for mother and baby, avoiding pulmonary aspiration, hypoxia, uterine atony and haemorrhage and providing good operating conditions, but it is a technique *for the skilled anaesthetist only*.

In conclusion, the safety of any method of analgesia or anaesthesia depends upon the skill of the administrator and on the facilities available. All methods cannot be made available everywhere. The first step towards effective analgesia in labour is taken in the education of the patient antenatally. Analgesia in labour should always start by the use of simple methods, which, if correctly used, can be very effective. Clinicians should offer to their patients only those methods which are SAFE in the situation in which they work.

INDICATIONS FOR OPERATIVE DELIVERY

For the purposes of this short book, it is considered more valuable to discuss the indications for the common operations practised in British obstetrics rather than to give comprehensive descriptions of operative technique which is best learnt by apprenticeship to a master. Details of operations will receive brief mention only.

Episiotomy
This is the most widely practised operation in obstetrics and in some hospitals is almost universal in primigravidae. Its proper performance is important to mother and child and its skilful repair is essential for safety and comfort in the puerperium.

Elective episiotomy is indicated in the following patients:

1. Where the baby is thought to weigh under 2·5 kg.
2. In those who have had a previous third-degree tear or extensive perineal repair.
3. In hypertensive and cardiac patients, to shorten the second stage of labour.
4. Where the breech presents.
5. In all operative vaginal deliveries.

Every effort must be made to anticipate the need for episiotomy, particularly in primigravidae, but situations will arise where emergency episiotomy is indicated – e.g. fetal distress or impending perineal tear.

Important points in the technique of episiotomy and its repair
1. When the head distends the perineum at the height of a contraction but still recedes between contractions, the perineum is infiltrated along the line of the intended episiotomy with 10 ml prilocaine (Citanest) 1·0 per cent.
2. Between contractions, the perineum is distended with two fingers and the open episiotomy scissors are placed in position. When the head advances on to the perineum one decisive cut is made, commencing the incision in the midline.
3. Wherever possible, the repair should be done in operating theatre conditions with full sterility and a good light.

4. The repair should be made under local analgesia – a further 10 ml of 1 per cent prilocaine can be given if necessary.
5. The repair should be made in layers, special attention being paid to securing the apex of the vaginal incision.

Complications of episiotomy
1. *Haemorrhage.* Postpartum haemorrhage may arise from failure to secure bleeding vessels, particularly at the vaginal apex. The vagina may fill up with blood so that the extent of the haemorrhage may not at first be apparent.
2. *Haematoma and bruising* of the perineum may be due to faulty technique but seems to be difficult to prevent in some cases.
3. *Infection and wound dehiscence* may result in weeks in hospital. Careful antiseptic and aseptic technique can usually prevent this. It is generally better to await granulation than to resuture.

Forceps delivery
Modern obstetrics should have little place for the 'difficult' forceps delivery. Difficulties should be anticipated and a timely resort made to Caesarean section in some cases.

The simplest general rule is that when the fetal head is visible at the vulva the case is likely to be a simple one and can be started under pudendal block or other suitable regional analgesia, but when the fetal head is not showing and particularly when some of the head is palpable above the pelvic brim, the delivery may turn out to be extremely difficult and hazardous. In these latter circumstances the obstetrician must ask himself three questions:

1. Is immediate delivery necessary?
2. Is the cervix fully dilated?
3. Is cephalo pelvic disproportion present?

The most important question is the first and if the answer to it is 'No' then a little time may be taken for the head to descend and a potentially difficult case may be transformed by nature into an easy one.

Conditions necessary for forceps delivery
1. The cervix must be fully dilated.
2. The presentation must be suitable – i.e. the vertex, face, or aftercoming head.
3. The head must be engaged.
4. There must be no obstruction to delivery at or below the level of the head.

5. The membranes must be ruptured.
6. Uterine contractions must be present.
7. The bladder and bowel should be empty.
8. Effective analgesia or anaesthesia should be given.
9. In most cases, an episiotomy should be made.

If these well-known conditions are observed the patient will be safeguarded from the trauma of an injudicious operation, and the inexperienced obstetrician will be safeguarded from dangerous errors. Observation of these conditions is much more important than the choice of any particular type of forceps.

Common indications for forceps delivery

Prolonged second stage of labour. If the cervix has been fully dilated for half an hour and no advance has been made the probable need for forceps delivery should be considered. In the presence of adequate uterine contractions and particularly if these are being stimulated by an oxytocin drip, few patients benefit from being left in the second stage for more than one hour.

The obstetrician must decide how long it is advisable for a particular patient to remain in the second stage and arbitrary times have really little significance. For example, any but the shortest of second stages may be too long for the woman with hypertension or heart disease.

Thought must also be given to the cause of the long second stage and here the following classification, no less valid for its antiquity, is helpful.

1. Faults in the powers – e.g. inefficient contractions may require oxytocin; patients who have had epidural block may be unable to push.
2. Faults in the passages e.g. prominent coccyx, narrow subpubic angle, rigid perineum.
3. Faults in the passenger – e.g. occipito posterior position or transverse arrest. In this context, the vital importance of diagnosing the position of the fetal head before applying the forceps (and therefore knowing the direction for rotation and traction) cannot be over-emphasised. William Smellie pointed out that the forceps should always be applied over the child's ears and observance of this simple rule will save much blood, sweat and tears.

Fetal distress. Objective evidence of this in the form of continuous fetal heart recording and fetal blood sampling is very helpful. If the fetus has been acidotic in the first stage or has been showing Type two dips on heart monitoring, preparations for forceps delivery should be made as soon as the second stage is reached. Interpretation of the signs of fetal distress can, however, be very difficult and the dangers of too early intervention, already mentioned, must be borne in mind.

'Trial of forceps' should always be performed by an experienced obstetrician in an operating theatre with all preparations made for Caesarean section. It is a potentially dangerous procedure because once the forceps is applied there is a temptation to use too much force. The occasions for its use should be few. If definite disproportion is present Caesarean section should be the primary treatment. Forceps delivery should only be considered in borderline cases. The most usual indication for trial of forceps is where the fetal head is in the occipito posterior position, perhaps rather deflexed and rotation above the level of the ischial spines is necessary. In these circumstances the obstetrician should be prepared to perform Caesarean section if a gentle attempt at rotation and forceps extraction fails.

Vacuum extraction

The technique required for vacuum extraction is different from that of forceps delivery and it can only be learnt in practice.

Indications for vacuum extraction

1. As an alternative to forceps delivery. Vacuum extraction is an elegant alternative to low forceps delivery under local anaesthesia and is often more comfortable for the patient as the vagina and perineum are not distended by the forceps blades. The object in applying traction with the instrument is to imitate the normal mechanism of labour, altering the direction of traction as the head extends. In simple cases the duration of traction is short and with skill and gentleness there is no damage to the baby: the cranium is not compressed as it sometimes is with the forceps and no marks are left on the face.

   For some cases in which rotation of the fetal head is required the vacuum extractor also has advantages and may, in experienced hands, be better than manual rotation or Kielland's forceps but such cases have to be chosen with care. Rotation occurs when the head is brought down on to the pelvic floor. When there is delay in the delivery of a second twin who presents by the vertex the vacuum extractor may be the ideal instrument, being sometimes much preferable to internal podalic version.

2. Where delivery is indicated late in the first stage of labour, with the cervix more than 6 cm dilated. Here the vacuum extractor can sometimes be dramatically successful but these are just the cases which require most skill and judgement and where the risk to the child is greatest. Misuse of the vacuum extractor in those circumstances can be a disaster. Trouble arises when obstetricians who have not had extensive practice in the method in easy cases encounter a patient who seems suited for delivery by vacuum extraction while still in the first stage – and then find themselves undertaking a difficult delivery with an instrument they do not fully understand.

The cup must be carefully applied so that cervix is not included. Traction must then be at right angles to the surface of the cup. Prolonged application should be avoided. If there is no progress within 20 minutes the procedure should be abandoned.

Before applying the vacuum extractor in the first stage, the obstetrician must ask himself:

1. Is delivery necessary now?
2. Is vacuum extraction the safest, best and quickest way for mother and baby?

The maternal risks of vacuum extraction are minimal. They are certainly less than those of Caesarean section. The main fetal risk is of scalp trauma: the small oedematous 'chignon' of scalp which the instrument causes disappears rapidly, but misuse can result in haematomata and lacerations which may be very serious.

Caesarean section
Caesarean section is being increasingly practised in Britain. A few years ago the Caesarean section rate in most maternity hospitals was around 7 per cent: now figures of 10 per cent are quite frequently reported. This increased incidence seems to stem from a number of reasons:

1. Greater readiness to perform repeat Caesarean section in patients previously delivered in this manner. This is related to modern limitation in size of families.
2. More sections are being done for malpresentations, particularly breech.
3. Antenatal and intrapartum fetal monitoring has resulted in more sections being done in the fetal interest.

In many cases the indications for Caesarean section are multiple, a combination of factors influencing the welfare of mother and child leading to the decision.

Caesarean sections may be *elective* operations, in which a decision is made to deliver the patient this way before labour starts, or they may be *non-elective*, generally the result of some complication arising during labour.

Indications for elective Caesarean section

1. *Previous Caesarean section*. A history of two previous sections is considered an absolute indication for delivery by repeat section. Vaginal delivery after one Caesarean section, performed for a non-recurrent indication, is often practicable and safe provided the case is managed in circumstances where a resort to repeat Caesarean section can easily be made. However, there is an increasing tendency to deliver by repeat section if the patient has a history of one previous Caesarean section and some complicating factor in the present pregnancy – e.g. twins, unstable lie.

2. *Placenta praevia*. All except the most minor cases of placenta praevia are now commonly delivered by Caesarean section because of the risk of haemorrhage to both mother and child. Before proceeding, every attempt should be made to make the diagnosis certain, e.g. by ultrasonic placentography and if necessary by vaginal examination under anaesthesia in theatre. The timing of delivery should be 38 weeks unless haemorrhage makes earlier delivery imperative.

3. *Cephalo-pelvic disproportion and contracted pelvis*. These cases, common when Caesarean section first became popular, are now unusual as indications for primary elective section in Britain. When a minor degree of disproportion is suspected neither the patient nor her baby is put at risk by allowing labour to progress for at least a few hours: with the use of oxytocin to produce effective uterine action and epidural block to give relief of pain, such cases often turn out to be surprisingly normal.

4. *Tumours in the pelvis*, such as an ovarian cyst or cervical fibroid.

5. *Previous repair operations*. A history of a Manchester repair with amputation of the cervix, a repair of any kind resulting in a successful cure of stress incontinence or the repair of a vesico-vaginal fistula are indications for elective section.

6. *Severe pre-eclampsia or eclampsia* may be an indication for elective section but the risks of the operation should be weighed against the possible efficacy of other methods.

7. *Placental insufficiency.* Babies whose growth has been shown by the usual monitoring tests to be severely retarded, may not stand up to the anoxia accompanying uterine contractions and may best be delivered by section. The timing of delivery requires great judgement and the possibility of congenital fetal anomaly as a cause of the growth failure must be borne in mind.

Indications for non-elective Caesarean section

1. *Failure to progress in the first stage of labour.* The active management of labour, using oxytocin to stimulate contractions and recording cervical dilatation graphically on the partogram, often results in failure to progress being highlighted at an earlier stage than formerly. None the less, the decision to perform a section remains a serious one and should only be taken by a senior obstetrician.

2. *Fetal distress.* These words are emotive and many sections have been done allegedly in the fetal interest on inadequate clinical evidence. Continuous fetal heart monitoring and fetal blood sampling make the situation clearer. The significance of abnormal signs must be weighed carefully against the possibility that delivery might take place in a short time if labour is rapidly progressive.

3. *Intrapartum haemorrhage* and some cases of *abruptio placentae* occurring before labour and with the fetal heart still present may be successfully managed by Caesarean section. This is a controversial subject because of the lack of objective evidence. Experienced obstetricians sometimes manage such cases vaginally, also with success.

4. *Malpresentations in labour*, particularly transverse lie, may be most safely delivered by section. There is little place for such procedures as internal podalic version unless the baby is thought to be pre-viable.

5. *Prolapsed cord.* This may occur at amniotomy or during labour and if the baby is alive and the cervix not fully dilated, Caesarean section should be done.

Type of operation

The lower segment operation is almost universally performed and a low transverse (Pfannenstiel) incision can also be used in the abdominal wall in most instances.

Classical Caesarean section may be indicated (rarely) in the following circumstances:

1. Difficulty and danger in getting access to the lower segment due to adhesions or fibroids.
2. Some cases of impacted transverse lie where extraction through the lower segment might lead to tears and haemorrhage.

Complications of Caesarean section

1. *Death.* This is dealt with in the section on maternal mortality. The maternal mortality associated with (but not necessarily directly due to) the operation is about 1 in 1000. This is about 10 times the mortality from vaginal delivery.

2. *Haemorrhage.* Even uncomplicated Caesarean section is associated with a blood loss of about a litre. Haemorrhage at the time of operation is usually due to (a) tears in the lower segment (b) failure of the uterus to retract, which may be aggravated by the type of anaesthetic.

3. *Pulmonary aspiration* and other complications of general anaesthesia. An increase in the use of epidural block where possible is recommended to avoid these.

4. *Thrombosis and embolism.* Figures for fatal pulmonary embolism show little improvement. The case for the use of prophylactic anticoagulants remains unproved. The use of a lateral tilt during the operation to take pressure off the great veins and ambulation as soon as possible after operation seem sensible measures.

5. *Paralytic ileus.* Prompt treatment by intravenous drip and gastric suction will help to minimise this serious complication.

6. *Sepsis.* If the patient has had pyrexia during labour or if the membranes have been ruptured for more than 24 hours, antibiotics (e.g. cephaloridine 1 G bd) should be given prophylactically. Swabs from the uterus should be sent for bacteriological examination. Similarly, in the puerperium, adequate bacteriological examination should precede any treatment and warning signs of infection should not be ignored.

7. *Wound haematoma.* This is sometimes extensive and may be associated with such a degree of anaemia as to require blood transfusion. Locally, it is best left to discharge and if the Pfannenstiel incision has been used, the wound usually heals well eventually without resuture.

MANAGEMENT OF THIRD STAGE OF LABOUR AND POSTPARTUM HAEMORRHAGE

Conduct of normal third stage

Delivery of placenta and membranes by maternal effort
Syntometrine 1 ml (containing ergometrine 0·5 mg and syntocinon 5 units) is given intramuscularly with the delivery of the baby's anterior shoulder. The purpose of giving syntometrine routinely is to combat atony of the uterus, not to hurry the third stage.

1. A bowl (the anatomically shaped Murdoch bowl is best) is placed against the perineum to catch all blood, so that the loss can be accurately recorded.
2. The ulnar border of the attendant's left hand is placed on the uterine fundus to observe retraction.
3. The signs of placental separation and descent are awaited. These are:
    a. Fundus is harder, rounder, more mobile and rises.
    b. Cord lengthens.
    c. There may be slight gush of blood from vagina.
    d. Placenta may be seen at vulva.
    e. Placenta may be felt in upper vagina and cervix on a sterile vaginal examination.
4. When the uterus is firmly contracted and the placenta is considered to be separated, the patient is instructed to bear down to try to expel the placenta, the abdominal wall being supported by the flat of the attendant's hand.
5. The placenta is received into both hands and the membranes eased out with an up and down movement.
6. The fundus is massaged and any blood clot expelled from the vagina.

Delivery of placenta and membranes by controlled cord traction (Brandt-Andrews manoeuvre)
This more active management of the third stage may be preferred in patients who have had induced or augmented labour and who are on oxytocin drip. Ergometrine 0·25 mg should be given intravenously with the birth of the anterior shoulder in these cases.

1. Having confirmed retraction of the uterus, the fundus is held behind the span of a pronated hand placed behind the symphysis pubis. The cord is grasped with the other hand and is put on the stretch.

2. The retracted uterus is then pushed firmly upwards, towards the patient's head, while constant steady tension is maintained on the cord in a downwards direction. The aim of the technique is to effect delivery of the placenta mainly by upward displacement of the uterus: traction on the cord merely helps to lift the placenta out of the vagina.
3. The fundus is massaged and any blood clot expelled.

Management of third stage haemorrhage

The procedures which have been described for delivering the placenta are designed to stimulate uterine activity in the third stage, to observe the signs of uterine retraction and to deliver the placenta in an atraumatic manner. In most cases these are effective techniques for preventing third stage haemorrhage.

If, despite their observance, excessive blood loss (i.e. more than 300 ml) occurs before delivery of the placenta, the objects of treatment should be:

1. Make the uterus retract. This can be done by massaging the fundus or by external bimanual compression. All clot should be expelled. A further dose of ergometrine should be given.
2. Empty the uterus. One further attempt at Brandt-Andrews or Crede's manoeuvre may be justified but manual removal may be necessary.
3. Replace lost circulating volume. This can be done rapidly with Ringer Lactate, Haemaccel or plasma while blood is being brought or cross-matched.
4. If manual removal is decided on, the uterus must be kept firm until the patient is in theatre, which should not be long. Anaesthetists are sometimes unwilling to induce general anaesthesia for manual removal until cross-matched blood is available, but delay may sometimes increase the danger to the patient.

Causes of postpartum haemorrhage

The causes of haemorrhage in the third stage and haemorrhage after the delivery of the placenta are often the same and they will be considered together here.

Haemorrhage may be atonic or traumatic.

Atonic postpartum haemorrhage
This is due to a failure of retraction of the uterus associated with such factors as:

1. *Retained products of conception.* In the third stage this is the

placenta itself. After delivery of the placenta it may be a retained placental fragment or even membranes.

2. *Overdistension of the uterus* as in hydramnios.

3. *Large placental site*, as in multiple pregnancy, where over-distension may also be present.

4. *Antepartum haemorrhage*. Placenta praevia may be associated with a failure of retraction of the placental site in the thin lower segment. In abruptio placentae, blood often infiltrates the uterine muscle (Couvelaire uterus) and this may interfere with retraction. In severe cases a coagulation defect may develop.

5. *Prolonged labour* is one of the textbook causes of postpartum haemorrhage. Its elimination by the use of oxytocin should reduce postpartum haemorrhage.

6. *Multiparity*. With successive pregnancies, the amount of fibrous tissue in the uterus increases and although uterine action may be very efficient in the first and second stages, retraction is sometimes poor. The 'grand multipara' is gradually disappearing from British obstetric practice.

7. *Fibroids* may interfere with retraction and sometimes cause severe postpartum haemorrhage.

8. *General anaesthesia*, particularly with halothane which is a uterine relaxant. Every attempt should be made to restrict the use of general anaesthesia to patients who really need it. If general anaesthesia is necessary a technique which minimises the risk of atonic haemorrhage should be used. Deliveries under epidural block are associated with less blood loss than those under general anaesthesia.

Traumatic postpartum haemorrhage

If bleeding continues despite firm uterine retraction the cause is some trauma to the genital tract which must be explored thoroughly in theatre to detect the bleeding site.

1. *Vaginal lacerations*. Bleeding may be coming from the apex of the episiotomy cut or from separate lacerations in the vagina. Sometimes the use of Kielland's forceps for rotation results in lateral or anterior vaginal lacerations.

2. *Laceration of cervix*. This is more common on the left side, perhaps because right occipito posterior position is more common that left. The whole circumference of the cervix must be inspected carefully grasping each area with sponge forceps and proceeding round it in an anticlockwise direction.

3. *Ruptured uterus*. This may be quite obvious, there being an

extension upwards of a cervical tear or a hole through a previous Caesarean section scar. If there is doubt whether the uterus is ruptured and if the patient's condition is deteriorating, laparotomy should be performed.

4. *Broad ligament haematoma*. External bleeding may be slight in these cases but a mass in the broad ligament (generally the left) will be palpable on bimanual examination. Management should be conservative as the condition is usually self-limiting and will resolve.

Management of postpartum haemorrhage
There are four principles which should be employed together:

1. Resuscitate the patient by the correction of hypovolaemia – preferably with blood.
2. Make the uterus retract – by ergometrine, massage, bimanual compression.
3. Empty the uterus ⎱ This means exploration of the genital tract
4. Repair any tears ⎰ – in theatre if possible.

If the patient is not in hospital the Flying Squad should be used to resuscitate her in her home and send her into hospital with a drip running and doctors and nurses in attendance. It is doubtful whether such procedures as manual removal of the placenta should be undertaken in the patient's home in an urban environment in Britain.

Inversion of the uterus
This is probably the most acute emergency in obstetrics. Its cause is obscure – all cases cannot be blamed on cord traction or mishandling of the uterus. If the uterine fundus turns inside out and appears at the vulva, it must be replaced INSTANTLY before there is time for spasm to occur for this will prevent replacement.

The patient with an inverted uterus becomes severely shocked and the situation is made worse by the haemorrhage which usually accompanies the inversion.

If immediate manual replacement is not successful the inversion should be reduced under general anaesthesia either manually or using a hydrostatic method, filling the vagina and uterus with warm sterile liquid. In occasional cases of partial inversion, laparotomy with division of the constricting ring may be necessary.

Secondary postpartum haemorrhage
This is a serious complication whose risks are sometimes underestimated.

Secondary postpartum haemorrhage is fresh bleeding from the genital tract anytime after the first 24 hours after confinement until the 6 weeks of the puerperium are completed. It is commonest between the 8th and 14th day after delivery. Any fresh bleeding in the puerperium is abnormal. Bleeding may at first be slight but the patient's general condition deteriorates more rapidly than would be expected from the amount of blood loss.

Active treatment – i.e. blood transfusion and exploration of the uterus to remove any small pieces of placenta or membranes – is indicated in all but the mildest cases. When the bleeding has been only slight, ultrasonic examination should be performed to identify any retained products.

In some instances no tissue is found in the uterus and the bleeding is then usually ascribed to infection.

If secondary postpartum haemorrhage recurs after curettage the situation becomes dangerous. The uterus should be *firmly* packed with gauze: this generally controls the bleeding. If it does not, or if bleeding recurs on removal of the pack 24 hours later, hysterectomy may be indicated.

3

Postnatal care

THE PUERPERIUM

Principles of management during the normal 'lying-in' period
(i.e. while the patient is in hospital)

Rest
The puerperium is a time of physical and psychological readjustment. It should begin with rest and adequate rest should be ensured throughout. Rest does not mean inactivity.

1. A good sleep on the first night is essential. Most patients will benefit at this time from an analgesic and hypnotic, e.g. pethidine 100 mg intramuscularly and nitrazepam 5 mg by mouth. This will relieve the pain from the perineal wound and will ensure that she starts the first full day of the lying-in period refreshed by sleep.
2. A happy atmosphere in the ward. This depends on the attitude of the nursing staff. The patient should feel relaxed, cared-for and able to turn to doctors and nurses for advice.
3. The patient should stay in hospital long enough to benefit from rest. The usual lying-in period is from 6 to 8 days. Patients who seek early discharge are sometimes those who will benefit least from it. It is difficult to provide in the home anything approaching the nursing care available in hospital. Relief from domestic chores and responsibilities is essential. One of the objects of antenatal education should be to explain the purpose and value of the week in hospital after delivery.
4. Not only should the patient be given a good sleep at nights (with the baby being removed to the nursery if necessary) but she should have a set rest hour in the afternoon. Doctors and nurses should recognise that she has a busy schedule, with baby care, visitors etc., and the rest hour should be sacrosanct.

Getting to know and care for the baby

1. Rooming-in is practised in most maternity hospitals. It cuts down the risk of neonatal infection and puts mother and baby together in natural circumstances. Sometimes mother and baby have to be separated because the baby is in the special-care nursery on account of prematurity or some other complication. Mothers may find this painful but being allowed to visit the baby and having the opportunity to talk to the Paediatric Staff usually reassures them.

2. The baby is bathed by the nursing staff when it is a few hours old to remove vernix, meconium and blood. The cord is cut short, tied and dressed with spirit. Thereafter the baby has no further complete bath until the day before discharge when the mother does it herself.

3. The mother does all the nappy changing herself and cleans the baby's bottom each time. The cord is treated with spirit and the baby is 'topped and tailed' and powdered twice a day – again by the mother. The nursing staff should supervise these processes in the early days.

Breast feeding. Mothers wash their own breasts. If the nipples are crusted the nurses help the mothers to bathe the crusts off. Nurses assist the mothers in the early stages to fix the baby on the breast. The baby is put to the breast at the age of six to eight hours and thereafter four hourly, for three minutes on each side, gradually increasing the time to seven or ten minutes on each side. After feeding the mothers apply their own nipple dressings.

Bottle feeding. Most hospitals have prepared feeds which can be used by the mothers. At the Queen Mother's Hospital in Glasgow a 'ready to feed' system is used and a four hourly routine is soon established.

Suppression of lactation. The main point about this is that oestrogens should be avoided because of the risk of increasing thrombo-embolism. The use of firm binders, diuretics and analgesics provides satisfactory treatment for engorged breasts.

Return to normal activity

1. Mothers are allowed up to the toilet within the first 24 hours.
2. They have a bath on the second day and are up for meals.
3. Bidets with running water sprays are used freely to cleanse the perineum. This greatly increases comfort and mobility.
4. No perineal or abdominal dressings are usually necessary.
5. Mobility is increased daily and the mother is soon quite active,

up and about, caring for her baby, having meals with the other patients, receiving visitors etc.

6. The physiotherapist should help the mothers by deep breathing exercises, perineal exercises and leg exercises. In the early days this is best done by a personal ward round by the physiotherapist. Later, mothers can attend classes in groups.

Observations by medical and nursing staff to detect any complications
1. Temperature and pulse are taken twice daily.
2. The blood pressure should be recorded once a day.
3. Involution of the uterus is recorded daily.
4. The lochia and perineum are inspected daily.
5. The haemoglobin level should be checked on the third or fourth day.
6. The nursing staff should check the state of the breasts while assisting with feeding.
7. Bowel and bladder function should be checked. It is the usual practice to give suppositories on the second day or third day if the bowels have not moved.
8. The patient's mental attitude and her reaction to caring for her baby and competence in doing it, should be noted.

Puerperal complications

Thrombosis and embolism
This is the main cause of death in the puerperium, as is discussed in the section on maternal mortality. A disturbing feature of the deaths from pulmonary embolism is that nearly half of them seem to have been preceded by warning signs, which if acted upon might have prevented the death.

1. Aetiological factors in puerperal thrombo-embolism are stasis of blood (which may be aggravated by antenatal bed rest or lack of activity in the lying-in period), infection, anaemia, pressure on leg veins during vaginal delivery or Caesarean section and the use of oestrogens to suppress lactation which produces increased coagulability of the blood.
2. Superficial venous thrombosis. This is often localised to a varicose vein in calf or thigh which becomes hard, reddened and tender. It is seldom associated with deep venous thrombosis, although signs of this must be looked for. It can be treated with local applications (e.g. Kaolin poultice), analgesics and rest from weight-bearing but active leg movements while in bed. The foot of the bed should be raised.

3. Deep venous thrombosis occurs in two forms – *ileo femoral thrombosis* and *phlebothrombosis of the calf*.

Ileo-femoral thrombosis, which gives rise to phlegmasia alba dolens or puerperal 'white leg' – fortunately rare now – is segmental in nature and may extend from the internal iliac vein as far down as the profunda femoris. It is usually of infective origin, in association with pelvic sepsis.

Phlebothrombosis of the calf is more common. Clotting occurs in the venous sinuses within the soleus muscle and thrombosis spreads to involve the popliteal vein.

Diagnosis of deep venous thrombosis: (a) *Clinical* – a complaint of pain in calf, tenderness on deep pressure, pain in the calf on dorsiflexion of the foot (Homan's sign) and swelling of the leg is the classical clinical picture but the trouble is that not all patients with deep thrombosis develop these signs.

(b) *Venography (phlebography)* may be done by the injection of a radio-opaque dye into a vein on the dorsum of the foot. It is a difficult technique and requires expertise to get good results but is probably worthwhile doing if the patient is suspected of having a pulmonary embolism and clinical evidence is unconvincing.

(c) I^{125} *labelled fibrinogen* can be given and the legs scanned the following day for thrombi.

(d) *Ultrasonic doppler effect* has been used to detect blood flow and therefore patency of major veins.

Treatment of deep venous thrombosis. The objects of treatment are:

1. To prevent further clot formation.
2. To prevent pulmonary embolism.
3. To relieve the symptoms.
4. To prevent residual disability.

All of these may be achieved by the timely intravenous injection of heparin which is the safest, quickest acting and most certain of the anticoagulant drugs. It inhibits the action of thrombin on fibrinogen and prolongs the clotting time. It also has a vasodilator effect. Prompt treatment may cause dramatic relief of symptoms. The initial dose is usually 15 000 units, followed by 10 000 units 4 to 6 hourly. If pulmonary embolism is suspected 25 000 units should be given as the first dose. Any puerperal patient may bleed and treatment with heparin has the great advantage that its action can be reversed by giving protamine sulphate 5–10 ml of 1 per cent solution.

It is the risk of bleeding that makes some clinicians doubtful about the role of oral anticoagulants such as warfarin whose action is not reversible.

The real problem is the difficulty of diagnosis for there is hesitancy in employing potentially dangerous methods of treatment unless the diagnosis is certain.

Puerperal pyrexia

A pyrexia of 38° or more is viewed as a sign of infection until proved otherwise. Most puerperal infections are endogenous i.e. arising from the patient's own body, chiefly gram-negative organisms from the bowel.

A search for the diagnosis should be made in the following 5 sites:

1. *The genital tract.* The lochia should be inspected, the uterus carefully palpated (it may be tender), perineal and abdominal wounds inspected and a cervical swab taken for bacteriology.
2. *The urinary tract.* Urinary infection is common in the puerperium but is usually of a mild nature with pyrexia, tachycardia and some dysuria and frequency. The classical picture of pyelonephritis with rigors, loin pain etc. is seldom seen. A mid-stream specimen of urine should be sent for bacteriological examination from all cases of puerperal pyrexia.
3. *The respiratory tract.* The common cold, influenza or bronchitis may be the cause of the fever. Streptococcal sore throat was associated with puerperal sepsis in the past but is now fortunately rare. None the less, throat swabs should be examined in all cases of puerperal pyrexia.
4. *The breasts.* Simple engorgement of the breasts may be associated with a rise in temperature. Gentle expression of the breasts by pump and treatment with diuretics may be necessary. If there is localised reddening of the breast with pain and tenderness immediate chemotherapy may abort the infection. Cephaloridine 2 g followed by 1 g b.d. should be given. Breast abscesses are seldom seen in maternity hospitals as they usually occur after the 10th day. Most breast infections are preventable by antenatal preparation of the breasts and the satisfactory establishment and maintenance of lactation.
5. *The legs should be examined.* Phlebothrombosis is not an infection but may be a cause of pyrexia.

Secondary postpartum haemorrhage

This has been dealt with in the section on postpartum haemorrhage.

Psychiatric disorders

Anxiety and depression are parts of normal life and it is not suprising that a great emotional event like childbirth should be followed by a psychological reaction.

A certain amount can be done in the prophylaxis of puerperal depression by an understanding attitude by the hospital staff.

1. Antenatal education classes instructing patients about childbirth; discussion forums with husbands present; visits to various departments of the hospital.
2. The patient should, if possible, know personally some of the team who will look after her in labour and should be able to discuss anxieties with them antenatally.
3. Husbands should be encouraged to help and sustain their wives during labour.
4. No woman should be left alone during labour.
5. Gentleness, understanding and a readiness to respond to questions during labour and delivery is important.
6. The woman should be informed, as reassuringly as possible, about the condition of the baby as soon as birth takes place.

Efforts like these build up a feeling of confidence between the patient and the hospital staff and remove much of the fear of being alone among strangers at the emotional crisis of birth. The feeling of confidence will encourage free communication about anxieties in the lying-in period.

Normal emotional reactions to childbirth. These include:

1. Feeling of depression, usually on third or fourth day – 'the blues'. The tension, excitement and emotional relief of the birth are over. Tiredness and physical discomfort now contribute to the feeling of depression. Tears for trivial reasons are common. Adequate rest and sleep is important at this stage and the patient soon recovers.
2. Anxiety about the baby. All mothers are anxious in case their babies are abnormal and anxiety is emphasised if mother and baby are separated for medical reasons – e.g. prematurity.
3. Grief in the event of a stillbirth, neonatal death or birth of an abnormal infant. If the baby dies it is usually best to send the mother home as soon as possible, but only after giving her and her husband as adequate an explanation as possible in the circumstances. An abnormal child who survives may be rejected by one or both parents or contrarily become the focus of attention to the detriment of brothers and sisters. In any event a long period of adjustment lies ahead.

Abnormal reactions to childbirth: (a) *Depressive psychoses* are the commonest form of serious mental illness in the puerperium. The clinical picture may be very varied. The patient may appear confused and probably does not sleep. She may dwell on the pain of labour or her own inadequacy. She may imagine her child is abnormal and that the staff are not telling her about it. She may fear she will injure her baby. If she shows any tendency to injure the baby it should be removed.

(b) *Schizophrenia* may appear in the early puerperium, particularly in those who have a previous history. The woman's behaviour may then be completely irrational.

Treatment of puerperal mental disorders. If the patient behaves in a frankly abnormal manner, seems unusually depressed or does not recover rapidly from depression, the advice of a psychiatrist should be sought. There is no place for amateurism at this stage any more than there is in an operating theatre.

Emergency drug therapy may include chlorpromazine (Largactil) 25 to 75 mg or trifluoperazine (Stelazine) 0·5 to 2 mg by intramuscular injection, but it is really more advisable that the psychiatrist should see the patient first and then prescribe the drugs.

THE NEWBORN CHILD

Resuscitation of the newborn

A generally accepted resuscitation procedure is as follows:

1. Clear the pharynx, mouth and nostrils by suction.
2. Lay the child head sloped downwards, on the 'Resuscitaire' or other suitable table.
   Do not put child's head up until respiration begins.
3. Supply oxygen by mask placed above baby's face.
4. If child is limp, stimulate movement by flicking soles of feet with finger.
5. If child responds by crying normally he is put head upwards and further oxygen is given until respiration is clearly established.
6. If the child does not improve, remains limp and does not breathe after three minutes, 15 mEq of sodium bicarbonate is given into the umbilical vein to correct acidosis.
   If respiratory depression can be attributed to morphine or pethidine 0·5 mg nalorphine is injected into the umbilical vein.
7. If child fails to respond the trachea is intubated under direct vision and positive pressure lung inflation is employed.

Examination of the newborn baby

The following examination should be made in all cases:

1. Check identity of baby and see that name tapes are in position.
2. Examine the head for caput, cephalhaematoma or moulding.
3. Look at general facial contour.
4. Look for cleft palate.
5. Inspect the ears.
6. Make sure arms are fully mobile and that there is no dislocation or paralysis. Count the fingers.
7. Examine the spine for evidence of spina bifida.
8. Examine the abdomen for liver enlargement or other palpable abnormality.
9. Check the anus is patent – this can be done by taking temperature per rectum.
10. Examine the feet for mobility and to exclude talipes.
11. Perform Ortolani's test for congenital dislocation of the hip which, briefly, is as follows:
    The baby is placed on his back: the knees are fully flexed and the hips flexed to a right angle. The baby's thighs are then grasped in both hands and abducted. In congenital dislocation of the hip the femoral head suddenly slips forward into the acetabulum with a distinctly palpable 'click'.

Common neonatal problems

Neonatology is a vast subject in its own right and the paediatrician has some justice in considering obstetrics to be just a branch of it – 'antenatal paediatrics'. Obstetrician and paediatrician should work as a team, with close contact to discuss all problems.

No attempt will be made here to do more than mention a few of the neonatal problems which the obstetrician encounters in the course of his own work.

Prematurity

This is the greatest neonatal problem of all and if the obstetrician could prevent it perinatal mortality would be much reduced.
Causes of prematurity are:

1. Unexplained. More than half the cases come under this heading. Poor social circumstances and poor diet are associated with prematurity but the way in which they operate is not clearly known. Premature labour may begin after rupture of the membranes: this may be due in some cases to cervical incompetence.

2. Twins. Careful antenatal management with periods of admission to hospital when indicated can cut down the risk of prematurity.
3. Hydramnios – often associated with fetal abnormality as well as prematurity.
4. Maternal pyrexia. Any severe pyrexial illness – e.g. pyelonephritis, pneumonia – may result in premature labour.
5. Trauma. A blow on the abdomen or external cephalic version may sometimes cause premature labour.
6. Abdominal operations during pregnancy – especially appendicectomy.
7. Pregnancy complicated by some condition which makes early delivery necessary (e.g. pre-eclampsia, placenta praevia). This is 'Iatrogenic prematurity'.

Every attempt should be made to prolong the pregnancy until the baby has the best chance of survival. The lecithin/sphingomyelin ratio in the liquor may be helpful.

Prevention and management of premature labour. Antenatal care will prevent some cases especially those with a previous history. Early cervical suture for cases of cervical incompetence and periods of rest and observation in hospital for those with an unexplained history may be helpful.

If premature labour begins spontaneously the decision has to be taken whether to give drugs in the attempt to stop it. In general, if the baby is 34 weeks mature and particularly if the membranes are ruptured, there seems little point in prolonging the pregnancy for a mere few days. At an earlier stage, however, when the risk of prematurity is greater drug treatment is worth attempting. Drugs used to arrest premature labour include:

1. Isoxsuprine produces uterine relaxation by direct stimulation of the β-adrenargic receptors of the myometrium. It also causes tachycardia and vasodilatation.
2. Orciprenaline ⎱
3. Ritodrine ⎰ these are newer β-receptor stimulants
4. Alcohol. Intravenous infusion of alcohol was reported on favourably at first but it is an unpleasant form of treatment for the patient.

None of the above drugs seems to be particularly certain in its action and their value is doubtful.

5. Salbutamol is a β-agonist. It may have a more selective action on uterine muscle than some of the other drugs and clinical trials are encouraging. Salbutamol, like other drugs with similar

action, produces tachycardia and its administration may need to be stopped if the maternal pulse rate exceeds 140 a minute or if the patient has tremors or palpitations. An intravenous infusion of salbutamol in a strength of 10 μg per ml is given in increasing dosage until contractions have ceased or until it has to be abandoned, because labour is progressing despite treatment, or side effects are developing. If treatment is successful in stopping contractions, the infusion rate is gradually reduced over the next 12 hours. Treatment with oral salbutamol tablets 4 mg four times daily is then continued for a week.

Complications of prematurity. Respiratory distress syndrome, the most dangerous of these, which may end fatally with intraventricular haemorrhage, presents the following clinical features:

1. Expiratory grunting.
2. Tachypnoea – more than 60 a minute.
3. Inspiratory recession of chest wall.
4. Cyanosis unless oxygen is given.
5. Characteristic X-ray changes – particularly the 'air bronchogram'.

The treatment of respiratory distress syndrome is by biochemical correction of acidosis and supportive measures such as oxygen, warmth and humidity.

Some cases have recently been treated by artificial respiration using continuous positive or negative airways pressure. (CPAP and CNAP). These methods are still at the experimental stage.

Other complications of prematurity include sepsis, jaundice and cold injury, all of which will be mentioned in connection with the neonate in general.

Neonatal hypoglycaemia
Profound hypoglycaemia, associated with symptoms such as fits and apnoeic attacks is associated with brain damage. This is preventable if every infant at risk has a blood sugar test at birth. The 'Dextrostix' screening test is easy to perform on all babies in the special care nursery. Babies particularly liable to hypoglycaemia include:

1. Small for dates babies. Early feeding should be given, intravenously if necessary.
2. Babies of diabetic mothers – often very hypoglycaemic at birth but blood sugar may rise spontaneously. If not, intravenous glucose should be given.

3. Babies with Rhesus Iso-immunisation.
4. Asphyxiated babies.

Hypocalcaemia
Plasma calcium is lower in babies fed on cow's milk. Fits occur typically between the ages of 5 and 8 days. The serum calcium is less than 4 mEq/l. Treatment is with a low phosphate milk (human milk or SMA) and oral supplements of calcium lactate.

Infection
Cross infection occurs from infant to infant. The umbilical stump is an important reservoir for organisms, particularly staphylococci and it is important to keep it dry and clean.

Epidemics of staphylococcal and intestinal infections occurred when babies were crowded together in communal nurseries but now that rooming-in has been almost universally established and nursing handling reduced to a minimum, these have greatly decreased. The simple and universal rule is that everyone who touches a baby washes his hands with soap and water before touching the baby and again after touching the baby.

Any case of neonatal sepsis, however minor, should be isolated. Specific infections worthy of note are:

1. Viral infections. Maternal virus infections may lead to fetal anomalies and to neonatal illness with jaundice, hepatospleno-megaly, thrombocytopaenia and anaemia.
2. Bacterial infections. Staphylococcal and streptococcal infections can be prevented by avoiding unnecessary handling and contact with other babies as mentioned, also by using hexachlorophane on the skin.
   Pseudomonas aeruginosa is a difficult organism to detect and treat. It lurks in water and may contaminate instruments.
   Antibiotic treatment with a combination of ampicillin and cloxacillin is the most popular for most infections while a combination of carbenicillin and gentamycin is effective against pseudomonas.

Jaundice
Important causes of jaundice are prematurity and Rhesus iso-immunisation but the commonest type seen in the lying-in ward is the so called 'physiological jaundice'. In any baby the bilirubin level rises for a few days before conjugation becomes efficient: about the 3rd or 4th day jaundice may become visible. The serum bilirubin should be estimated in all cases and if it continues to

rise, the baby should be transferred to the paediatric department for treatment. This will consist of adequate feeding and may include the use of phenobarbitone which increases bilirubin conjugation in the liver and phototherapy, because blue light will convert bilirubin in the skin to harmless pigments and produces lower plasma levels. Plasma levels of unconjugated bilirubin greater than 20 mg/100 ml are toxic to the brain and produce the staining of the basal ganglia known as kernicterus.

The most rapid and reliable method of reducing serum bilirubin is by exchange transfusion and this should be undertaken in all severe cases.

Haemorrhage
1. A baby may be anaemic at birth due to intrapartum blood loss. This possibility should be borne in mind in cases of twins, antepartum haemorrhage and Caesarean section. Transfusion may be necessary.
2. Bleeding due to haemorrhagic disease of the newborn occurs between the third and fifth days and is usually gastro-intestinal. It is more common in breast fed babies who have less Vitamin K. The treatment is an intramuscular injection of Vitamin K (phytomenadione).
3. Bleeding from the umbilical stump may be due to inefficient clamping.
4. Cephalhaematoma or scalp haemorrhage may result from obstetric trauma. It is sometimes severe enough to require transfusion with fresh frozen plasma or blood.

Cold injury
Newborn babies are liable to injury and even death from hypothermia. Birth asphyxia and prematurity increase the hazards. The baby is drowsy, anorexic with red skin, he feels cold and there may be oedema. Very careful rewarming over a prolonged period is necessary.

In hospital, babies are at risk from cold when being resuscitated, bathed, X-rayed or otherwise exposed naked, or when being transported about the hospital. Adequate clothing including covering the head with a bonnet is necessary particularly for the premature baby.

In an incubator, a small premature baby needs a high temperature which would be too hot for a term infant.

A cot-nursed infant needs a room temperature of 26°C and a cot-nursed 1500 g baby needs a room temperature of 30°C.

THE POSTNATAL EXAMINATION

Much was written in the past about the value of the postnatal examination, mainly about such subjects as the correction of retroversion and the treatment of cervical erosions. An advance from this mechanistic point of view has taken place, but the postnatal clinic is all too often a neglected area. Not all patients will attend it. Some prefer not to come at all. Every effort should be made to see the following groups:

1. Those who have lost their babies from stillbirth or neonatal death or abortion.
2. Those who have had operative deliveries – particularly Caesarean section.
3. Those who have had complications of pregnancy which necessitated antenatal admission.

The objects of the postnatal examination
1. To assess the woman's general health. A general physical examination, as deemed necessary including haemoglobin and blood pressure recordings, should be done.
2. To examine the breasts and discuss any feeding problems.
3. To make a pelvic examination
   a. to check that the perineum is well healed and there is not likely to be dyspareunia;
   b. to confirm involution and the normality of the uterus and adnexa;
   c. to take a cervical smear.
4. To discuss the prospects for future pregnancies. Ample time should be taken for the woman to bring out any anxieties, however irrational they may be, and to discuss these more calmly than it is possible to do in the lying-in ward. She may want to know e.g., 'Shall I need a Caesarean section for my next baby?' or 'Why was my baby premature?' or more poignantly 'Why did my baby die?'. The obstetrician, probably knowing the patient personally and with the full case record before him, is in a unique position to deal with these questions. This is the most important part of the postnatal examination.
5. To discuss family planning. This subject should have been raised while the patient was still in the lying-in ward and her feelings and intentions ascertained and recorded in the case sheet. It should be discussed again at the postnatal examination and definite plans should be made at this time. Prescriptions

for the contraceptive pill can be given and arrangements made for the insertion of an intrauterine device or for laparoscopic sterilisation. The patient is much more likely at this stage to have her mind clear about which method she wants than she was during the emotionally unstable week after the birth. The obstetrician's duty is to make sure that, with his agreement, the plan she favours is carried out.

4

Complications of pregnancy

ABORTION

Abortion means termination of pregnancy, whether spontaneous or induced, before the 28th week, that is, before the fetus is viable.

Abortion in its various forms is probably the greatest problem in obstetrics and gynaecology and it is the greatest cause of maternal death. Sepsis of a particularly dangerous and overwhelming nature is the most important cause of death from abortion.

Incidence

It is often stated that the incidence of spontaneous abortion is about 15 per cent of pregnancies, but it is extremely difficult to get reliable figures. More than half of those aborting spontaneously do so before the 12th week. The incidence of induced abortion (legal or illegal) varies according to the social customs and laws of different countries.

Causes of spontaneous abortion

1. *Chromosomal abnormality*

Chromosomal abnormality is responsible for about 1 in 5 cases of spontaneous abortion. As genetic studies become more widespread, information on these cases is accumulating.

Abortion in these circumstances is a beneficial process and represents a form of natural selection.

2. *Endocrine defects*

Endocrine defects have long been postulated as causes of abortion, but evidence remains inconclusive. Biochemical evidence of hormone deficiency is merely a sign that the function of the trophoblast is inadequate and replacement therapy does not seem to correct this dysfunction.

3. *Abnormal implantation*
There is evidence that abnormal sites of implantation (e.g. over the os) may be associated with an increased abortion rate.

4. *Multiple pregnancy*
The larger the number of fetuses, the greater the tendency to abortion. This may be due to overdistension of the uterus.

5. *Uterine causes*
   a. Cervical incompetence – may be congenital or acquired due to trauma of previous operations or births. Typically, cervical incompetence causes mid-trimester abortion preceded by premature rupture of the membranes.
   b. Double uterus – in its various forms, this is the result of anomalies of fusion of the Mullerian ducts. The greater the degree of duplication, the more normal is pregnancy likely to be.
   c. Fibroids may sometimes distort the uterine cavity and produce abortion but pregnancy proceeds without interruption in many women with multiple fibroids.

6. *Infections*
   a. Any severe pyrexial illness may cause abortion.
   b. Specific infections such as syphilis, brucellosis and listeriosis have been suggested as causes of abortion. Conclusive evidence on these subjects is lacking.

7. *Poisons*
A number of systemic poisons may cause abortion, particularly cytotoxic drugs.

8. *Radiation*
As with cytotoxic drugs, abortion following radiotherapy is sometimes encountered during treatment for cancer.

9. *Dietetic*
The most important dietetic factor which has been implicated as a cause of abortion is folic acid. There is no evidence to suggest, however, that administrations of folic acid will prevent abortion.

10. *Immunological*
The rejection of the pregnancy by the mother for immunological reasons would seem theoretically a likely cause of abortion. There is little information of practical value on this subject so far. The

commonest immunological problem encountered in pregnancy is Rhesus iso-immunisation and here abortion sometimes results.

Clinical varieties of abortion

The process of abortion can be represented in the following diagram:

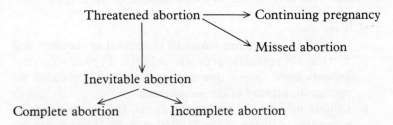

1. *Threatened abortion*
This is characterised by:

    a. Bleeding after amenorrhoea.
    b. Usually no uterine contractions and no pain.
    c. Cervix remains closed.
    d. Uterus is expected size for dates.

2. *Inevitable abortion*
This is associated with:

    a. Increased bleeding – clots often passed.
    b. Uterine contractions and pain.
    c. On examination, cervix is found to be dilating and products projecting. In some cases the conceptus has passed entirely into the cervical canal which is distended ('cervical abortion').

3. *Complete abortion*
    a. Whole conceptus is expelled.
    b. Uterus contracts down to near normal size.
    c. Bleeding stops.

4. *Incomplete abortion*
This is often the result of interference (legal or illegal).

    a. Part of conceptus has been passed or has been removed.
    b. Bleeding continues and may be severe.
    c. Vagina may be full of clot and patient may become shocked before adequate treatment is started.
    d. Infection may supervene.

5. *Missed abortion*
This means the retention in the uterus of a dead conceptus.

   a. Uterus fails to grow.
   b. Symptoms and signs of pregnancy – e.g. breast enlargement – will regress.
   c. Brown vaginal discharge may be present.

Investigation and treatment of abortion

1. *Threatened abortion*
When a woman gives a history of painless fresh vaginal bleeding after an interval of amenorrhoea the most likely diagnosis is threatened abortion.
The clinician must ask himself several questions:

   a. Is she pregnant?
   b. Is the pregnancy intrauterine?
   c. Is it a viable pregnancy?
   d. Is there any evidence of the abortion becoming inevitable?

If the answer to the first three questions is 'yes' and the answer to the fourth is 'no' the patient can be treated on traditional lines with bed rest and mild sedation.
The diagnosis is made and the questions answered as follows:

   a. *Is she pregnant?* General symptoms and signs of pregnancy and the finding of a soft cystic uterus, enlarged to a size consistent with the dates, on bimanual examination. Pregnosticon test positive.
   b. *Is the pregnancy intrauterine?* Findings as above suggest intrauterine pregnancy but the possibility of ectopic should be remembered in all cases. In ectopic pregnancy pain before bleeding is usually characteristic and there is considerable tenderness on pelvic examination.
   c. *Is it a viable pregnancy?* This question cannot be answered clinically in the early months, but ultrasonic examination has a unique value in outlining the fetus and detecting the fetal heart action from 6 weeks onwards. If no fetus is seen and no fetal heart detected, it is likely that either the patient is not pregnant or has a non-viable pregnancy – a 'blighted ovum'. However, it is best to repeat the examination at an interval of at least a week before abandoning an attempt to conserve the pregnancy.
   d. *Is there any evidence of inevitable abortion?* Painful uterine

contractions, increased bleeding and dilatation of the os usually mean inevitable abortion but it is worth observing the patient closely for a little while to see if these features disappear.

It has already been said that the treatment of threatened abortion is rest and sedation. The object of treatment is to encourage continuance of the pregnancy. There is no scientific basis for hormone treatment. Progestational agents may cause virilisation of a female fetus and in any case appear to be completely ineffective.

The most important thing the obstetrician can do is to encourage a feeling of confidence in the patient. Ultrasonic examination is a great help because if the fetus is outlined and the heart found to be beating there is good cause for optimism. On the other hand, if the fetus is dead or is not present as in the 'blighted ovum' the patient may be saved weeks of false hope and unnecessary anxiety.

The psychological aspect of threatened abortion should never be minimised. It is a most upsetting experience and is usually followed by anxiety throughout the rest of the pregnancy about the normality of the child. The patient needs understanding and support from her doctor to cope with these problems.

2. *Inevitable abortion*

While the object of the treatment of threatened abortion is to conserve the pregnancy, when abortion becomes inevitable the aim should be to aid the process and produce a complete abortion so that the risks of haemorrhage and sepsis can be cut to a minimum.

It is always worthwhile making a vaginal examination on any patient who is admitted with a threatened abortion and subsequently has further bleeding and pain. If this is not done a woman with an inevitable abortion may bleed substantially without the diagnosis being made.

On examination it is sometimes possible to remove digitally the whole conceptus from the cervical canal or from the vagina. If this is not possible, give morphine 15 mg with syntocinon 5 units and ergometrine 0·5 mg as an intramuscular injection. This will sometimes produce complete abortion. If there is any suspicion that the abortion is incomplete and particularly if there is further bleeding, exploration of the uterus should be done in theatre.

3. *Complete abortion*

If the abortion is complete no specific treatment is necessary, but there is often some doubt about the diagnosis. This can be resolved by·

   a. Ultrasonic examination for retained products.
   b. Curettage of the uterus.

If the ultrasonic examination shows an empty uterus, curettage may be unnecessary.

4. Incomplete abortion
This is the most dangerous type of abortion, particularly as it is often associated with previous interference and the patient may face the double danger of:

   a. Haemorrhage.
   b. Sepsis.

The treatment is to empty the uterus so that the retained products which are the potential cause of further haemorrhage and also the focus of infection can be removed.

   a. Resuscitate the patient by correcting hypovolaemia.
   b. Remove all clot and tissue from vagina.
   c. Ergometrine 0·5 mg.
   d. If there is pyrexia or other evidence of sepsis give an effective dose of antibiotic e.g. cephaloridine 2 g.
   e. Evacuate the uterus in theatre as soon as possible.

When doing this operation remember:

   a. The uterus may be already damaged by previous interference.
   b. It is very easy to perforate the uterus with instruments. If it is possible to remove products of conception digitally, this should be done before using sponge-holder or curette.

As has already been stated, sepsis of a particularly dangerous and overwhelming nature is the chief cause of death from abortion. Patients with septic incomplete abortion are particularly liable to develop endotoxic shock from Gram-negative organisms and this possibility should always be kept in mind. Profound hypotension, out of proportion to the amount of blood loss, is usually the first sign. Treatment of endotoxic shock which is discussed in more detail on pages 177–180, is a complex matter and is best undertaken in an intensive therapy unit to which the patient should be transferred if it is within reasonable distance. The main principles of treatment are:

   a. Correction of hypovolaemia – with blood if necessary – central venous pressure monitoring is essential.
   b. Intensive antibiotic treatment.

    c. Give large doses of hydrocortisone – 1 G initially and 3–4 G in 24 hours.

    d. Correct hypoxia. Oxygen should be given – if necessary by artificial ventilation. Blood gases should be monitored.

    e. Correct metabolic acidosis.

    f. Watch for signs of coagulation disorder.

    g. Watch for renal failure – treat with dialysis if necessary.

4. *Missed abortion*

The diagnosis can be confirmed by *negative pregnancy urine tests* and, more certainly, by *ultrasonic examination* which will show no evidence of fetal heart action and perhaps no fetus at all – as in the 'blighted ovum'. It is as well, however, to be cautious before proceeding to uterine evacuation because both tests can sometimes be misleading. The patient will not come to any harm from waiting a few days until the diagnosis is certain.

    a. If the uterus is less than 12 weeks' size it can usually be evacuated instrumentally without danger but if the patient will accept a more conservative policy there is much to be said for it as operation always involves risks of haemorrhage and sepsis.

    b. If the uterus is more than 12 weeks' size it is preferable to start the abortion process with prostaglandin and syntocinon.

    c. If the products of conception are retained for more than 3 weeks, clotting factors should be checked as a coagulation disturbance may be present, although this is rare.

Habitual abortion

This term is used when a woman has had three or more consecutive abortions.

Causative factors are found in less than 50 per cent of cases but some middle trimester abortions are due to cervical incompetence, in which case treatment by cervical suture in one of its various forms is rational.

However most patients with histories suggestive of habitual abortion do not fall into this group and for them rational and effective treatment is seldom available.

The following facts should be ascertained:

1. Is the history true?
2. Are hospital records available for inspection?
3. Was a fetus seen?

4. Were chorionic villi seen on histological examination of uterine curettings?
5. At what stage of gestation did the abortions occur?
6. Is there a history of previous trauma or operations on the uterus?
7. Is there a history of previous illness (e.g. viral infection) in association with the abortions.

Careful investigation of the history may reveal that the patient has not been pregnant at all but has been having episodes of metropathia haemorrhagica which masquerade as abortions. The problem then is one of infertility.

If a pregnant woman is proved to have a true history of early abortions, it is best to employ simple measures of rest and reassurance combined with evidence that the present pregnancy is proceeding normally. This can best be done by repeated ultrasonic examination to show growth and persistent fetal heart action. Controlled trials have shown that hormone therapy seems to be ineffectual. If the patient is not pregnant, endocrine investigations regarding ovulation may be indicated. Hysterography to exclude abnormal uterine shape may also be useful.

Induced abortion
Induced abortion may be legal or illegal. The United Kingdom Abortion Act of 1967 states that abortion can be performed provided two doctors are satisfied that there is risk to the life or health of the mother, or that there is a high risk that the child will be malformed.

It was also stated that social factors and the welfare of existing children should be taken into account when assessing risk to health. This legislation has been interpreted with great variability and consequently abortion is performed more often by some doctors than by others.

Any abortion performed by badly trained persons in inadequate premises is particularly dangerous because of:

1. Haemorrhage.
2. Trauma.
3. Infection.

Methods of inducing abortion
1. Instrumental dilatation and curettage. This is generally safe up to 10–12 weeks, but the earlier it is done the better.
2. Suction curettage. This is also a safe method in the early weeks.

Careful maintenance of apparatus is essential. Positive instead of negative pressure in the apparatus has caused death.

3. Injection into the uterine cavity of hypertonic solutions has a high risk of complications and has largely been replaced by prostaglandins.

4. Prostaglandins. The extra-amniotic administration of prostaglandins by a Foley catheter inserted through the cervix is a safe and effective way of inducing abortion, particularly in the middle trimester. The rate of infusion of prostaglandin is controlled by an automatic pump. Syntocinon is often given in addition and seems to have a synergistic effect. Curettage for retained products is often required after abortion by this method.

5. Abdominal hysterotomy is a certain method of terminating pregnancy but involves the risks of major surgery and also increases the risk in subsequent pregnancies. It is practised much less since prostaglandin termination has become available.

6. Hysterectomy may be justified in some instances where the patient desires sterilisation or where a subsequent pregnancy would involve great risk. It may sometimes be preferable to the fashionable procedure of combining vaginal evacuation of the uterus with laparoscopic tubal diathermy which has led to deaths from intravascular injection of carbon dioxide.

Every case in which abortion is decided upon must be reviewed critically to assess which is the safest method for the patient. Large series of 'outpatient' abortions have claimed that risks are minimal, particularly in early pregnancy, but deaths from legal abortion do occur and have risen to equal those now occurring from illegal abortion.

Legal abortion is further discussed on pages 164 to 169.

ECTOPIC PREGNANCY

Ectopic pregnancy is a comparatively common, dangerous and potentially fatal condition. In some of its forms it is very difficult to diagnose clinically. Laparoscopy is the chief diagnostic aid.

Aetiology

The most common form of ectopic (extra-uterine) pregnancy is tubal and the commonest site is the ampulla.

The cause is a partial obstruction of the Fallopian tube, insufficient to prevent spermatozoa from fertilising the ovum in the tube but sufficient to prevent the ovum passing through to the uterus. The commonest cause of this is *chronic salpingitis* due to:

1. *Gonorrhoea.* The incidence of ectopic pregnancy is greatest in those communities where gonorrhoea and pelvic inflammation are most common.
2. *Tuberculosis.* Tuberculous salpingitis generally causes complete tubal occlusion but this may partially resolve after treatment and the risk of ectopic pregnancy then increases.

Some cases of ectopic pregnancy may follow sterilisation operations or tubal surgery for infertility and occasional ones are due to rare congenital anomalies.

Pathology

1. The trophoblast, implanted on the tubal mucosa, erodes the tube wall. Intra-tubal or intraperitoneal bleeding occurs and as a rule the embryo then dies. The tube usually becomes a distended haematosalpinx, with varying amounts of bleeding from it.
2. Microscopically, chorionic villi are seen in the tubal wall and lumen.
3. The endometrium reacts to the hormonal stimulus of the trophoblast by converting itself into a decidua, which is generally cast off in pieces, causing the irregular uterine bleeding which is a symptom of ectopic pregnancy.

Tubal pregnancy may terminate in several ways and the clinical features will vary accordingly.

1. *Tubal rupture.* Trophoblast erodes through the tube causing massive and sometimes fatal haemorrhage.
2. *Tubal abortion.* The ovum separates from the wall of the tube and is gradually squeezed out the fimbriated end, from which bleeding takes place. The contractions of the tube during this process cause colicky abdominal pain.
3. *Pelvic haematocele.* Slow effusion of blood forms a large haematoma in the pouch of Douglas.
4. *Secondary abdominal pregnancy.* The placenta may gradually grow through the tube and find a secondary implantation in the abdominal cavity. There have been many fulltime abdominal pregnancies, some resulting in live births by abdominal section.
5. *Intraligamentary pregnancy.* Occasionally the products of conception may perforate the tube between the layers of the broad ligament and continue to grow there.

6. *Mummification of fetus.* If ectopic pregnancy is unrecognised the fetus may be retained in the abdomen. Fetal bones may eventually be discharged through the abdomen or rectum, or calcification of the fetus may occur.

Symptoms and signs

There are various clinical syndromes characteristic of ectopic pregnancy.

1. Sudden abdominal pain and collapse, accompanied by intense pallor (peripheral vaso-constriction), restlessness and shoulder-tip pain. This is the picture of massive intra-peritoneal haemorrhage. Vaginal bleeding is usually slight and there is sometimes no preceding amenorrhoea.
2. Chronic abdominal discomfort, occasional fainting, irregular vaginal bleeding or bloodstained discharge. This is the commonest and most treacherous type of case for the early symptoms may not be severe and may be mistaken for those of normal pregnancy, threatened abortion or pelvic inflammation. Delay in reaching the correct diagnosis may be dangerous or even fatal as a massive haemorrhage may supervene.
3. Pelvic swelling may be due to a haematocele.
4. Advanced abdominal pregnancy is a rarity but its possibility should occur to the doctor who notes any bizarre signs on antenatal abdominal examination.

The differential diagnosis of ectopic pregnancy can be very difficult, particularly in the chronic forms described under (2) above.

1. Pain usually precedes bleeding, unlike threatened abortion where bleeding comes first. Vaginal bleeding is usually slight in ectopic.
2. There is no marked pyrexia.
3. Vomiting is not a common factor.
4. Shoulder-tip pain is common.
5. Lower abdominal tenderness is usually present – not sharply localised.
6. Abdominal rigidity and guarding are unusual.
7. Extreme tenderness is often elicited on vaginal examination. Sometimes a tender pulsatile adnexal mass can be felt, but if the tube is ruptured there may be no palpable mass.

These features may help to differentiate ectopic pregnancy from such conditions as:

1. Pelvic inflammatory disease.
2. Acute appendicitis.
3. Uterine abortion.
4. Perforated peptic ulcer.
5. Acute urinary infection.

Diagnostic aids

Clinical diagnosis of a ruptured ectopic pregnancy with an abdomen full of blood is not difficult. Diagnostic aids are chiefly necessary in the more chronic cases.

Culdocentesis. Aspiration of blood from the posterior vaginal fornix.

Abdominal paracentesis. This is only of value when a considerable amount of blood has already accumulated in the peritoneal cavity.

Laparoscopy. This is the most valuable of all the diagnostic aids. If blood is seen in the peritoneal cavity, the diagnosis of ectopic pregnancy is almost certain and laparotomy should be performed. If no blood is seen the patient can be saved unnecessary laparotomy.

Pregnancy tests. Urine tests are of doubtful value. A negative test does not exclude the possibility of continued growth of the trophoblast and perforation of the tube.

Sonar. Ultrasonic diagnosis of ectopic pregnancy is difficult e.g., it may be impossible to tell difference between a tubal pregnancy and a corpus luteum cyst. The most useful application of sonar is in a case where an early *intrauterine* pregnancy, with positive fetal heart signs, can be clearly defined. This makes the diagnosis of ectopic pregnancy extremely unlikely.

Treatment

The treatment of ectopic pregnancy is laparotomy with removal of the affected tube and evacuation of blood and clot from the peritoneal cavity.

Resuscitation should be simultaneous with surgery. There is no point in delaying operation while blood is pouring into the abdomen.

The whole Fallopian tube should be removed, as attempts at conservation may merely allow the formation of another pregnancy in the remaining part of the tube.

Blood loss should be replaced by transfusion. Autotransfusion, by filtering and infusing into a vein blood removed from the peritoneal cavity has been useful where transfusion services are not available.

HYDATIDIFORM MOLE

Incidence: 1 in 2000 in Western countries: 1 in 200 in some Asian countries. It seems to be more common in elderly patients, particularly primigravidae.

Clinical features

1. Amenorrhoea and pregnancy symptoms followed by irregular vaginal bleeding.
2. Vomiting may be excessive.
3. Pre-eclampsia may occur at an unusually early stage in pregnancy.
4. Uterus usually bigger than dates would suggest, but in some cases it may be equivalent or smaller.
5. Fetal heart not heard.
6. Theca-lutein cysts in ovaries (due to excessive HCG stimulation) may be palpable.
7. Vesicles may be passed.
8. Urine pregnancy tests positive in high dilution (1 in 200 or more).
9. Sonar. Ultrasonic examination reveals typical 'snow storm' picture inside uterus. No fetus can be identified.

Pathology

Hydatidiform mole is due to cystic degeneration of the chorionic villi. The syncitium and Langhan's layers persist, but the mesodermal core of the villus undergoes myxomatous change and blood vessels disappear. The power to invade persists because trophoblastic elements are still there.

Hydatidiform mole can co-exist with a normal pregnancy as a form of twinning. Mole can also occur in a partial form, with a fetus present. This is a form of hyperplacentosis.

Risks of mole

1. Haemorrhage $\left.\right\}$ as in abortion
2. Sepsis
3. Toxaemia
4. Subsequent choriocarcinoma. Molar metastases occur in about 5 per cent of cases: these are apparently benign lesions. Choriocarcinoma follows mole in from 2 to 17 per cent of cases and is the main risk.

Management of mole

Once the diagnosis is made, the mole should be removed. This may be done by:

1. Prostaglandin (extra-amniotic) and oxytocin stimulation.
2. Suction evacuation.
3. Abdominal hysterotomy.
4. Hysterectomy.

If vaginal evacuation is performed it is desirable to do a repeat curettage in 10 days to make certain that all tissue has been removed.

Follow-up of mole

All cases must be carefully followed for evidence of persisting trophoblast.

Chorionic gonadotrophin (HCG) tests should be done at intervals. Radioimmunoassay is the best method.

Tests should be done every week until normal and then at monthly intervals for at least a year. During this time the patient should be advised to avoid pregnancy. If HCG levels are not normal 8 weeks after evacuation of a mole, chemotherapy should be started.

Choriocarcinoma

This disease was almost universally fatal in the past. It is now curable with chemotherapy. The main agent in treatment is the folic-acid antagonist, methotrexate. If treatment is begun within six months of the preceding pregnancy, the condition is probably always curable.

Treatment with methotrexate is hazardous and must be carefully controlled because the dose of folic-acid antagonist which will kill all trophoblast is close to the dose which will kill the mother by complete marrow suppression.

Methotrexate is sometimes used in combination with mercaptopurine – a purine and Vitamin B12 antagonist.

Cytotoxic therapy for choriocarcinoma is best performed in specialised units to which the patient can be conveniently transferred.

This subject is considered in further detail on pages 224–225.

ANTEPARTUM HAEMORRHAGE

Causes

Vaginal bleeding after the 28th week of pregnancy may be due to:

1. Placental separation
   a. Placenta praevia
   b. Abruptio placentae
2. Local causes
3. Uncertain cause

The last group of cases is numerically the greatest. In them the delivery is completed without the cause of the bleeding ever being clearly known.

1. *Placental separation*

a. *Placenta praevia*

If the placenta is implanted wholly or partly in the lower uterine segment, bleeding is almost inevitable as the lower segment stretches and the cervix is taken up. The clinical features are:

(i) Painless fresh bleeding for no apparent cause.
(ii) First incident of bleeding usually a slight one ('warning haemorrhage') but may be succeeded by massive haemorrhage.
(iii) Uterus is not usually tense or tender.
(iv) Presenting part is high and free or there may be a malpresentation.

Diagnosis of placenta praevia. All cases of antepartum haemorrhage should be viewed as being due to placenta praevia until proved otherwise. (This applies even to those in which the diagnosis of abruptio seems clinically obvious, for the two conditions may co-exist and it is unwise to perform a vaginal examination in such a case without theatre being set).

a. If it is obvious that delivery is urgently necessary, the diagnosis can be made by examination under anaesthesia with theatre set for Caesarean section.
b. If the haemorrhage is of minor degree, allowing time for investigation, placentography should be done. Numerous methods are available, including soft tissue radiography and arteriography but ultrasonic examination yields the best results. If a major degree of placenta praevia is clearly seen on ultrasonic examination, the eventual delivery should be

by Caesarean section without prior vaginal examination. If time is available, repeated ultrasonic examination may be done to confirm the diagnosis. It is sometimes found that, in the earlier months, the placenta appears to alter in position when weekly ultrasonic examinations are done. This is probably due to alterations in shape of the lower segment.

Treatment of placenta praevia. The conservative management originally advocated by Macafee is now universally employed. The patient is kept in hospital and an attempt made to prolong the pregnancy till 38 weeks. At this time the baby is mature enough to survive but after this time the risk of major haemorrhage is increased as labour may start. A desire to secure a mature baby should not blind the obstetrician to the maternal risk of recurrent haemorrhage and often it is this which determines the timing of delivery. All but the most minor cases of placenta praevia are now delivered by Caesarean section. Dangers during this operation include the risk of an adherent placenta (placenta praevia accreta) and the risk of continued haemorrhage from a poorly retractile lower segment. Packing the uterus may be effective for the latter, but hysterectomy should be considered before the patient's condition becomes desperate.

Modern management has produced good maternal and fetal results in placenta praevia but the condition still remains a major emergency and a potential cause of death.

b. *Abruptio placentae*
This mysterious condition, where there is premature separation of a normally situated placenta, remains completely unexplained, despite associations with:

(i) Hypertension and pre-eclampsia.
(ii) Anaemia and folic acid deficiency.
(iii) Multiparity.
(iv) Poor social conditions.

There is no doubt that the number of cases of abruptio placentae admitted to British maternity hospitals has fallen very greatly in association with better antenatal care, prophylaxis of anaemia and decreasing multiparity but major cases of abruptio can still occur in e.g., healthy young primigravidae, so the aetiology remains obscure.

The clinical features of a classical case are:

(i) Abdominal pain with or without vaginal bleeding (de-

pending on whether bleeding is 'mixed' or 'concealed').
The pain is sudden in onset and continuous in character: it is due to infiltration of blood between the uterine muscle fibres ('Couvelaire uterus').

  (ii) Rigid tender uterus: fetal parts difficult to feel.
 (iii) Fetal heart sounds absent.
 (iv) Hypovolaemic shock of varying degree – if the patient has previously been hypertensive, arterial blood pressure may be misleading.

Treatment of abruptio placentae. The principles of treatment are:

1. Resuscitate and apparently 'over-transfuse' the patient with blood. Blood loss is always more than is imagined. Central venous pressure should be used to monitor transfusion.
2. Test for and be prepared to treat clotting defect. Clotting tests should be done on the first specimen of blood taken for cross-matching and appropriate treatment instituted. If the condition is recent, fibrinogen deficiency may be the main feature and replacement of fibrinogen (e.g. 8 G) may be very effective.
3. Expedite delivery. Labour often starts spontaneously after abruptio placentae. Early delivery is desirable in all cases to reduce the risk of further bleeding. If the fetal heart is still heard there may be a place for Caesarean section. If the baby is dead, vaginal delivery after amniotomy is preferable. Syntocinon may not be necessary and should be used with caution as it may not be possible to monitor uterine contractions accurately. The patient should always be nursed on her side to avoid supine hypotension.
4. Watch for and be prepared to treat postpartum haemorrhage. Delivery of the baby may be followed by a massive retroplacental clot and an atonic postpartum haemorrhage. Ergometrine 0·5 mg should be given intravenously as the anterior shoulder is delivered.
   The most experienced person available should be present at the delivery in these cases as quick action may be necessary.
5. Watch for and be prepared to treat oliguria and renal failure. If intrapartum management has been effective adequate renal perfusion should have been maintained but the risk of renal failure should always be remembered. Serum urea and electrolytes should be estimated during labour and if urinary output is not adequate during the first 12 hours after delivery treatment should be started. Mannitol is often effective (with or without

a diuretic such as frusemide) in producing diuresis before renal pathology becomes established.

6. Treat anaemia in the puerperium. Despite apparently adequate blood replacement, many patients who have had abruptio placentae are found to be anaemic in the puerperium. Further blood transfusion may be necessary. Acute folic acid deficiency may occur and require treatment.

2. *Local causes of antepartum haemorrhage*

This is a comparatively small group of patients but if a local cause for bleeding is discovered the patient can sometimes be sent home or appropriate treatment started. Bleeding from local causes may occur spontaneously or after intercourse. Examples of local causes are:

a. Vaginitis – trichomonas or monilia.
b. Cervical polyp.
c. Cervical erosion.
d. Carcinoma of cervix.

With the exception of the last, which is rare, bleeding from these causes is of minor degree.

In any patient with *slight* antepartum bleeding it is desirable to pass a speculum (but not a finger!) into the vagina while bleeding is still present to see:

a. If there is a local cause.
b. If blood can be seen coming through the cervical os, in which case it can be assumed that the bleeding is intrauterine in origin.

3. *Antepartum haemorrhage of uncertain cause*

Most of the women who have vaginal bleeding in the last 12 weeks of pregnancy never have the cause discovered. In the past many of these cases were ascribed to 'revealed accidental haemorrhage' or 'marginal haemorrhage' but although such mechanisms may operate, it is difficult to justify these diagnoses when no evidence of placental separation can be demonstrated. It is better therefore to group such cases as being of 'uncertain cause'.

Every effort must be made to exclude placenta praevia in all cases.

It has been thought that antepartum haemorrhage of uncertain cause is dangerous because:

a. The placenta may have sustained damage leading to placental insufficiency.
b. A major haemorrhage may follow.

These arguments have been used to justify delivery in all cases at 38 weeks or sometimes earlier but there is little evidence to support them as results are likely to be good in any case once 38 weeks is reached.

The real risk of antepartum haemorrhage of uncertain cause is in association with *prematurity*.

If bleeding occurs and is followed by labour while the baby is still premature, the fetal mortality and morbidity is increased due to prematurity.

This is an important obstetric problem and management is unsatisfactory. The use of suppressants of uterine action such as salbutamol and ritodrine is of doubtful value in a patient who has had bleeding but if the baby is very premature and bleeding seems to be settling, they may be worthwhile, as may be the use of betamethasone in an attempt to accelerate lung maturation.

HYPERTENSION, PRE-ECLAMPSIA AND ECLAMPSIA

There have been few subjects about which so much has been written with so little precision. This is because there has been great difficulty in establishing agreed *definitions* about hypertension and pre-eclampsia and it is impossible to make valid international comparisons and, furthermore, the *cause* of pre-eclampsia remains unknown.

It is none the less true that hypertension in pregnancy is a major cause of maternal and perinatal death and therefore regular observation of blood pressure during pregnancy is a vital part of antenatal care. Good antenatal care and perhaps improved social conditions appear to be effective in producing a decline in the incidence of pre-eclampsia.

The following findings are generally accepted as normal during pregnancy.

1. Blood pressure should be below 140/90 mmHg. A slight drop occurs in both systolic and diastolic levels in mid-pregnancy.
2. Slight oedema is present in about two thirds of women at some stage in the last 3 months of pregnancy.

BUT proteinuria – NIL. The presence of protein in the urine should always be regarded as abnormal.

Classification of hypertension in pregnancy

Hypertension present before 24 weeks. This is usually classified as 'pre-existing hypertension' (except in rare cases like the acute pre-eclampsia syndrome associated with hydatidiform mole).

Pre-existing hypertension may be due to:

1. Essential hypertension.
2. Chronic renal disease.
3. Endocrine disorders (e.g. Conn's syndrome, phaeochromocytoma).
4. Connective tissue diseases.
5. Coarctation of aorta.

Hypertension noted after 24 weeks may be due to pre-existing hypertension (as above) or may be a new phenomenon – 'pregnancy-induced hypertension' or 'pre-eclampsia'.

A rise in blood pressure is the first sign of pre-eclampsia. The prognosis worsens as the blood pressure rises and is much worse if proteinuria (> 250 mg/l) is also present. Proteinuria heralds an increased danger to both mother and fetus in all cases.

The risk of pre-existing hypertension is increased when proteinuria appears ('superimposed pre-eclampsia') and the syndrome is then identical with that of pregnancy-induced hypertension.

Oedema is so common in late pregnancy as to be regarded as normal in itself, but the incidence and severity of oedema rises in the presence of hypertension and is often greatest when hypertension and proteinuria are both present.

Parturition has usually a striking effect on pre-eclampsia – blood pressure falls, oedema disappears and proteinuria clears, generally after a few days: but occasional cases of postpartum hypertension and even of eclampsia occur.

Factors which pre-dispose to pre-eclampsia

1. Parity – first pregnancy.
2. Age – older patients more at risk. (The severe cases sometimes seen in teenage girls are often associated with poor antenatal care.)
3. Obesity.
4. Pre-existing hypertension.
5. Multiple pregnancy.
6. Diabetes mellitus.
7. Rhesus iso-immunisation.
8. Hydatidiform mole.

Theories on the aetiology of pre-eclampsia

No attempt is made to list all the possible explanations of the 'disease of theories'. A few are as follows:

1. *Endocrine dysfunction.* Hypertension in Cushing's syndrome is

associated with excess glucocorticoid production from the adrenal and in hyperaldosteronism with excess mineral corticoids, but pre-eclampsia may occur after bilateral adrenalectomy so a pure adrenal cause seems unlikely. Excessive anti-diuretic hormone from the pituitary has also been postulated as a cause, but may be merely an effect of pre-eclampsia.

2. *Utero-placental ischaemia*
   a. Reduction in utero-placental blood flow may be mechanical as in the primigravida with her firm abdominal musculature or in the patient with an over-distended uterus as in multiple pregnancy.
   b. Vaso-active agents may be released into the maternal circulation, perhaps due to altered metabolism in the placenta: that the placenta plays an important role is suggested by the increased incidence of pre-eclampsia where there is excessive placental tissue (e.g. mole, Rhesus disease). Vaso-active agents may result in utero-placenta ischaemia and also in more general effects.

3. *Disseminated intravascular coagulation.* Widespread intravascular fibrin deposition has been shown in patients dying of eclampsia and it has been suggested that in pre-eclampsia there is a process of disseminated intravascular coagulation, possibly caused by the release of substances from the placenta. There is now a great deal of evidence to prove that there is a disturbance of intravascular coagulation in pregnancies complicated by hypertension and proteinuria but the relationship of this finding to the cause of pre-eclampsia is not clear. It is not known what initiates intravascular fibrin deposition. Treatment of severe pre-eclampsia with anticoagulants has, so far, been disappointing and is hazardous.

4. *Immunological disturbance.* It has been suggested that this theory is supported by the facts that pre-eclampsia is more common in first pregnancies, less common in consanguinous marriages and that fluorescent rhesus antibodies bind to proliferative vascular lesions of the placenta in erythroblastosis.

Pathology of pre-eclampsia

1. *Placenta.* 'Infarcts' have for many years been reported as typical of pre-eclampsia but some of these may not be true infarcts at all. Placental bed biopsies obtained at Caesarean section from patients with hypertension and proteinuria showed fibrinoid necrosis of decidual arterioles, and infiltration of damaged vessels with foam cells and round cells.

2. *Kidney.* There seems to be a specific glomerular lesion associated with pre-eclampsia. The glomeruli appear enlarged with swelling of capillary endothelial cells, thickening of basement membrane, hyperplasia of intercapillary cells and narrowing of capillaries.
   Electron microscopy confirms enlarged and cellular glomeruli; increased mesangium; fibrin in Bowman's space and in capillary loops.
   Similar changes have been found in the kidney in cases of abruptio placentae.
3. *Liver.* There is not a great deal of information on the state of the liver in pre-eclampsia but it is well known that subcapsular haemorrhages and periportal necrosis are associated with eclampsia.

Risks of pre-eclampsia to the mother
1. Eclampsia.
2. Cerebral haemorrhage.
3. Abruptio placentae.
4. Renal failure.
5. Risks associated with Caesarean section.

Risks of pre-eclampsia to the fetus
1. Intrauterine death.
2. Neonatal death and complications of prematurity (usually due to obstetric intervention necessary in the maternal interest).
3. Intrauterine growth retardation.
4. Possible physical and mental retardation associated with intrauterine malnutrition or gross prematurity.

Management of hypertension in pregnancy
1. Admit to hospital for initial assessment.
   a. To obtain frequent recordings of blood pressure and assess the severity of the hypertension.
   b. To investigate any possible underlying cause – e.g. chronic renal disease, phaeochromocytoma.
   c. To determine the maturity of the pregnancy by clinical and ultrasonic examination. This information is vitally necessary when assessing the timing of delivery.
   d. If the patient is already in the third trimester, to assess the function of the feto-placental unit by daily oestriol measurements and weekly ultrasonic cephalometry.

This initial assessment of hypertension is best performed in early pregnancy in cases of pre-existing hypertension and as soon as the blood pressure rises in pregnancy – induced hypertension. It puts the whole clinical picture into perspective. In many instances the blood pressure reaches normal levels within 48 hours.

2. If the blood pressure settles or does not rise above 150/90 mmHg, the patient can often be sent home and observed at fortnightly intervals, or more often if indicated, at the antenatal clinic. Readmission is indicated if:

   a. Blood pressure rises again.
   b. Proteinuria develops.
   c. There are symptoms of impending eclampsia.
   d. Marked alteration in weight; excessive weight perhaps indicating fluid retention and loss of weight indicating placental insufficiency.
   e. Signs of intrauterine growth retardation.
   f. Falling oestriol levels.

3. Hospital treatment of mild hypertension alone (i.e. diastolic blood pressure less than 100 mmHg). Rest in bed (but not complete immobility) combined with mild sedation may reduce the blood pressure and also, it is believed, help to nourish the fetus by increasing the feto-placental circulation.

4. Treatment of hypertension (Diastolic B.P. > 100 mmHg) and proteinuria. Conservative measures are tried first if the pregnancy is at less than 38 weeks. Bed rest and sedation (as above) are combined with a hypotensive drug such as methyldopa 250 mg thrice daily.

   If the pregnancy is 38 weeks mature there is no point in persisting with conservatism and induction of labour or Caesarean section should be performed as appropriate.

5. Treatment of severe pre-eclampsia or impending eclampsia. Conservatism has no place here. The pregnancy should be terminated. Management is on similar lines to that discussed below for eclampsia.

6. Treatment of eclampsia. Eclamptic fits are the sequel to uncontrolled pre-eclampsia. Warning signs are:

   a. Rapid rise in blood pressure.
   b. Headache.
   c. Visual disturbances.
   d. Abdominal pain.
   e. Vomiting.
   f. Twitching.

The principles of management of eclampsia are:

a. To stop the fits.
b. To prevent their recurrence.
c. To reduce the blood pressure.
d. To terminate the pregnancy.

If a patient has eclampsia at home she should be brought into hospital by the obstetric flying squad. The fits can be brought under control in the home by simple measures such as the injection of diazepam 10 mg intravenously. Blood pressure can be reduced by intravenous hydrallazine starting at 20 mg and increasing by 5 mg doses. An alternative anticonvulsant is chlormethiazole (Heminevrin) which can be given in an intravenous drip, but it has no hypotensive action.

On admission to hospital anti-convulsant therapy is continued and steps are usually taken to terminate the pregnancy.

Epidural block is a good method of controlling hypertension, relieving pain and allowing any necessary obstetric manipulations to be done with the minimum disturbance to the patient. Vaginal delivery can usually be achieved after amniotomy and intravenous syntocinon, but the induction-delivery interval should not be prolonged and Caesarean section should be considered in suitable cases.

Intensive anti-convulsant and anti-hypertensive therapy should be continued throughout labour and for about 12 hours afterwards, only being stopped when it is seen that the patient's condition is definitely resolving.

Renal failure should be anticipated by monitoring fluid intake and output, blood urea and urine urea.

If there is oliguria despite adequate hydration, renal failure should be suspected. Initial treatment should be with intravenous frusemide or mannitol.

Eclamptic patients should always be investigated for evidence of coagulation defect – e.g. low platelet count and 'burr cells' seen on blood film. If such a defect is found, specialised treatment may be advised by the haematologist.

Late results of hypertension, pre-eclampsia and eclampsia
It is important that patients who have had these complications attend for follow-up so that an attempt may be made to find out:

1. Whether pre-eclampsia predisposes to hypertension in later life.
2. Whether pre-eclampsia unmasks a latent tendency to hypertension (e.g. in the diabetic).

Most patients who have had pre-eclampsia are found to be normotensive when they attend for postnatal examination six weeks postpartum and their renal function is also unimpaired. It seems unlikely that pre-eclampsia is an important cause of latent hypertension. The chances are that they will not develop pre-eclampsia in a subsequent pregnancy but the risk of this is greater for patients who have had pre-eclampsia than for those who have never had it at all.

Recurrent pre-eclampsia may be a manifestation of chronic hypertensive disease which remains latent except during the stress of pregnancy.

RHESUS ISO-IMMUNISATION

Development of rhesus iso-immunisation

Rhesus immunisation can occur when red blood cells containing the Rh or D antigen enter the circulation of a woman who does not have this antigen on her red cells.

This may be caused by:

1. Incompatible blood transfusion. This causes multiple immunisation against D, C and E antigens.
2. Pregnancy with a rhesus positive fetus. The immunisation resulting from pregnancy is nearly always due to the D antigen alone. Rhesus positive red cells enter the maternal circulation at pregnancy or delivery. The risk of feto-maternal transfusion is increased by complications such as abortion, external cephalic version, antepartum haemorrhage, Caesarean section and manual removal of the placenta. Fetal cells can be detected in the maternal blood by means of the acid-elution technique – they can stand up to immersion in citric acid buffer whereas adult cells are eluted and appear on the blood film as 'ghosts'. The development of rhesus immunisation seems to depend on the volume of fetal cells transfused into the maternal circulation. A rhesus negative woman whose fetus is ABO incompatible is usually protected from immunisation because her anti A or anti B antibody will remove the A or B positive cells entering her circulation.
Rhesus immunisation is hardly ever found during a first preg-

nancy: it seems that the feto-maternal transfusion associated with delivery is necessary before the process starts.

10 to 12 per cent of women at risk develop antibodies 6 months after delivery and a further 10 per cent are found to have antibodies in a subsequent pregnancy.
Two types of antibodies are found:

a. Immunoglubulin M (IgM) antibody. Large molecule. Does not cross placenta.
b. Immunoglubulin G (IgG). Smaller molecule. Can cross placenta.

Prevention of rhesus iso-immunisation

Prevention is achieved by the injection of anti-rhesus immunoglobulin G after delivery. If the fetus is Rh positive and the mother Rh negative, but not immunised, this injection is given within 48–72 hours of delivery. The injected antibody causes the removal of any fetal red cells in the maternal circulation and is eventually itself destroyed by the normal process of protein breakdown in the body.

Anti Rh IgG is obtained from naturally immunised women by plasma phoresis, so its availability depends upon blood donations.

Effects of rhesus iso-immunisation

The effects on the fetus are:

1. Congenital haemolytic anaemia.
2. Hydrops fetalis.
3. Icterus gravis neonatorum.
4. Kernicterus.

The mechanism of production of these well known effects is briefly as follows. The removal of circulating red cells by haemolysis results in anaemia and hypoxia. Placenta hyperplasia occurs to increase oxygen transfer. If hypoxia persists the fetus develops cardiac failure with oedema and ascites – the syndrome of hydrops fetalis. Haemolysis of red cells results in a rise in unconjugated bilirubin which is mainly excreted into the maternal circulation by the placenta. Some bilirubin enters the amniotic fluid where its amount is an indication of the severity of the disease. After delivery the bilirubin cannot escape via the placenta and circulates in the infant causing jaundice – icterus gravis neonatorum – because the liver cannot conjugate the excessive amount of bilirubin in the circulation. High levels of bilirubin can cause damage to the basal ganglia of the brain – kernicterus.

Management of rhesus iso-immunisation

Aims of management are:

1. To deliver a live child.
2. To deliver as mature a child as possible.
3. To deliver a child who has avoided the most severe manifestations of immunisation such as hypoxia and hydrops fetalis.

It is obvious that the sooner the child is removed from its unfavourable intrauterine environment the sooner will it be possible to arrest the haemolytic process. The limiting factor is maturity.

Methods of assessing severity are:

1. Maternal antibody levels are only a rough guide.
   If the antibody titre rises to more than 1 : 8 by Coombs amniocentesis should be done.
2. Amniocentesis is the most useful method of assessing the fetal condition. Wherever possible the position of the placenta should be ascertained by ultrasonic examination before the needle is inserted into the uterus so that damage to the placenta can be avoided and the risk of feto-maternal transfusion minimised. Maternal venous blood samples are taken before and after amniocentesis to assess whether feto-maternal transfusion has occurred and, if so, its amount.
   Bilirubin in the amniotic fluid is estimated by spectro-photometry. A prediction is made on the basis of results previously obtained in large series of cases and plotted on a graph such as that devised by Liley. If the bilirubin level is high and the fetus is still too premature to deliver intrauterine, intraperitoneal transfusion of the fetus with rhesus negative blood should be undertaken. This procedure is done under X-ray screening and the amount of blood transfused is calculated according to the maturity of the fetus. The object of intrauterine transfusion is to act as a holding operation until the baby is big enough to deliver. Transfusions can be repeated at 2 or 3 week intervals. Intrauterine transfusion is not without risk and various fetal injuries and maternal complications including infection have been reported.
   By the time the pregnancy reaches 34–36 weeks the fetus is better to be delivered and further treatment undertaken in the

paediatric department. Prompt paediatric treatment is required for the seriously affected infant. Exchange transfusion remains the keystone of treatment but other measures such as correction of acidosis and the use of phototherapy with ultraviolet light may be required.

A small group of mothers whose previous histories of fetal loss from rhesus disease are particularly bad may be treated throughout pregnancy by repeated plasma phoresis of their own blood to wash out the antibodies. This is a very time-consuming and mentally stressful treatment and not all patients accept it easily. It requires to be done in a specially equipped centre. In desperate cases it has something to offer and is sometimes attended with success.

5

Diseases associated with pregnancy

HEART DISEASE IN PREGNANCY

Even in normal pregnancy there is a greatly increased burden on the heart. This is partly due to increased body weight associated with fluid retention of hormonal origin and the weight of the enlarged uterus, fetus and placenta but, more importantly, due to the circulatory adjustments which occur during pregnancy.

Haemodynamic changes in normal pregnancy

1. Blood volume increases from the 8th week to about the 36th week of pregnancy when it is about 35 per cent above the non-pregnant level. The plasma volume increases by 40 per cent approximately, whereas the red cell volume increases by 20 per cent approximately. There is a decrease in plasma volume near term resulting in a drop of about 15 per cent from the peak level of blood volume.

2. Cardiac output increases to about 30–40 per cent above the non-pregnant level by the end of the first trimester and only changes slightly thereafter. This early rise in output may be due to ovarian and placental hormones. No change is recorded in cardiac output if the patient is lying on her side, but output falls if measured in supine position after 32 weeks due to compression of inferior vena cava by the enlarged uterus. Most patients have an adequate collateral circulation by the para-vertebral veins but if collateral circulation is inefficient, supine hypotension results. Cardiac output rises further in labour due to increased stroke volume and is maximum just after delivery when there is a return of blood to the heart from the uterus and from the lower limbs due to the release of caval compression. Output returns to non-pregnant level by end of second week postpartum.

3. Heart rate increases only slightly during pregnancy.

4. Arterial blood pressure does not alter much during pregnancy.

5. Oxygen consumption increases in pregnancy although respiratory excursion is impaired in later weeks.

6. Blood viscosity decreases during pregnancy and this helps to compensate for the extra work the heart has to do.

Incidence of heart disease in pregnancy

This varies from place to place but at present is probably around 2 per cent. Most cases are still due to rheumatic heart disease but there has been a recent decline in rheumatic cases and an increase in the number of women with congenital heart disease who reach childbearing age. All patients who have had cardiac surgery are exposed to increased danger in pregnancy.

Diagnosis of heart disease in pregnancy

Early diagnosis is essential so that strict antenatal supervision can be given to all cardiac cases, because the main problem is the presentation of the cardiac patient in late pregnancy without adequate care. At the first antenatal visit the patient may give a clear history of cardiac disease or rheumatic fever but more often there is no such history and diagnosis may be very difficult. Functional heart murmurs are often difficult to distinguish from organic ones. Physiological murmurs are heard in about one third of all pregnant patients. Such murmurs are of ejection type and can be heard anywhere over the praecordium. Pan-systolic and diastolic murmurs always indicate organic heart disease. The louder an ejection murmur is, the more likely it is to be organic. Any patient with a cardiac murmur or a history of dyspnoea should be referred to a cardiologist. Many hospitals have a combined obstetric/cardiac clinic. Physician and obstetrician should assess possible complications in the light of patient's age, parity, previous medical and obstetric history and present clinical state and a strict policy of frequent antenatal visits laid down. Where necessary, patients should be admitted to hospital for further assessment.

Classification of heart disease

The most common convention is to classify cardiac cases according to the grades laid down by the New York Heart Association.

Grade I: signs of cardiac disease but no symptoms.

Grade II: signs of cardiac disease with slight limitation of activity.

Grade III: signs of cardiac disease with marked limitation of activity, symptoms arising on slight exertion.

Grade IV: signs of heart disease with the patient unable to carry out any activity without discomfort.

The patient's response to effort is a very important guide as to behaviour in pregnancy but this classification is open to criticism because all grades of heart disease are potentially dangerous. Any pregnant cardiac patient may be precipitated into congestive failure or acute pulmonary oedema by any cause of tachycardia and all are at risk from infection.

Complications of heart disease in pregnancy

The worst things that can happen are:

1. Acute pulmonary venous congestion leading to pulmonary oedema. This can be precipitated by onset of rapid atrial fibrillation.
2. Bacterial endocarditis. This remains a cause of maternal mortality and all potential causes of infection must be watched for. Antibiotic prophylaxis must be given to all patients with rheumatic or congenital heart disease.

Treatment of heart disease in pregnancy

Surgical

Mitral valvotomy. Mitral stenosis is still the commonest form of rheumatic heart disease encountered in pregnancy. Valvotomy during pregnancy should be avoided where possible as results are much better if performed when patient is not pregnant. It is practically never done now during pregnancy, certainly not in the later weeks when risk of operation is far greater than continuation of pregnancy.

Ligation of patent ductus. This operation could be performed during pregnancy if necessary but most patients with patent ductus are treated in childhood.

Termination of pregnancy. This is rarely required on cardiac grounds alone.

Medical treatment

Nearly all patients with heart disease can be satisfactorily managed during pregnancy by medical treatment alone. Frequent antenatal visits are required. Where possible, patients should attend fortnightly. If this is inconvenient, home visits by the general practitioner could be arranged. The following rules should be observed in all cases:

1. Adequate rest and sleep. 8 to 10 hours in bed at night and a mid-day rest of 2 hours. If patient cannot get adequate rest at

home, admission to hospital will be necessary. In many cases admission at some time between 28 and 32 weeks can be useful for joint assessment by the obstetrician and cardiologist. The medical social worker can often help in making necessary arrangements.

2. Avoidance of smoking.
3. Prevention and treatment of anaemia.
4. Dental care with antibiotic cover for any extractions.
5. Treat all infections as potentially dangerous. Antibiotics should be given freely but, even more important, patients should be admitted for proper diagnosis and assessment. Upper respiratory infections and particularly influenza may precipitate cardiac failure.
6. Oral diuretic therapy with potassium supplements for fluid retention where necessary, particularly for those with symptoms of pulmonary venous congestion or signs of pulmonary hypertension.
7. Digitalisation. It is not unreasonable to digitalise patients while still in sinus rhythm if there is thought to be a risk of atrial fibrillation developing e.g., patients with symptoms or signs of commencing pulmonary hypertension. In digitalised patients atrial fibrillation occurs at a lower rate and acute left heart failure is less likely.
8. Anticoagulants. The most likely reasons for giving anticoagulants are:

a. Prosthetic heart valves.
b. Rheumatic heart disease with atrial fibrillation.

The problem of transplacental passage of oral anticoagulants can be solved by substituting intravenous heparin (the large molecule of heparin does not cross the placenta) after 37 weeks or whenever delivery is thought to be likely. Patients with prosthetic valves should be advised to be sterilised because of the need for long-term anticoagulants.

Emergency management of acute pulmonary oedema
Diagnosis. Acute severe dyspnoea; may be haemoptysis with frothy sputum; moist sounds at both lung bases.

Treatment
1. Sit the patient up with legs over edge of bed.
2. Give oxygen (high flow, 8 litres/minute) by Hudson mask or similar apparatus.

3. Inject morphine 15 mg intramuscularly.
4. Give a diuretic, e.g. Frusemide 40 mg–80 mg intravenously.
5. If no improvement, perform venesection withdrawing 500 ml of blood. This is seldom necessary.

Induction of labour

It is preferable to admit the patient to hospital before labour starts. In general it is best to await the spontaneous onset of labour. Traditionally, induction of labour has been avoided because of the danger of introducing infection. Modern methods of induction have reduced the induction-delivery interval and, with it, the incidence of infection. Where a valid indication for induction exists it should be performed without hesitation. Antibiotics should be given to all cardiac patients in labour whether spontaneous or induced. Cephaloridine or cephalexin are suitable drugs because they are effective not only against the streptococcus but also against gram-negative organisms which are the most frequent pathogens in modern obstetric practice.

Management of labour

1. Relieve pain early and efficiently, e.g. by morphine 15 mg intramuscularly or by epidural block.
2. Keep the pulse rate down. If the pulse rate is around 80 per minute the patient is usually not in danger. A rise of pulse to more than 100 per minute must be viewed as a grave sign. Adequate relief of pain helps to keep the pulse rate down. If necessary, Digoxin should be used.
3. Keep the patient propped up or lying on her side in a comfortable position during labour.
4. Prevent infection by strict asepsis and antisepsis and by antibiotic cover.
5. Vaginal delivery is generally preferable to Caesarean section but no cardiac patient should be allowed to have a prolonged or difficult labour. If Caesarean section is necessary, it is better done early rather than late. Careful pre-labour assessment may result in some patients being delivered by elective Caesarean section.
6. Unless the patient progresses rapidly and easily to a spontaneous delivery, forceps or vacuum extraction should be employed in the second stage. Vacuum extraction can be done with the patient sitting up.
7. The third stage should be treated normally. It is preferable to give ergometrine than allow the patient to bleed in an un-

controlled manner. Ergometrine 0·25 mg given intravenously is usually efficient and safe but a careful watch should be kept for any signs of congestive failure in the third stage or immediately afterwards.

Puerperium

1. Sedation and careful observation in bed for 24 hours.
2. Early ambulation thereafter to avoid thrombo-embolism.
3. No contraindication to breast feeding in patients who can undertake normal activity without dyspnoea. Oestrogens should not be used to suppress lactation.
4. Watch for signs of infection. Always remember risk of bacterial endocarditis and the difficulty in diagnosing this condition. Blood cultures should be taken in the event of any pyrexia.
5. Before sending patient home, check that home conditions are adequate and that sufficient domestic help is available. The aid of the medical social worker should be sought.
6. Discuss contraception and sterilisation. If she decides on sterilisation give her a date for admission in about 8 weeks' time. This is preferable to performing sterilisation in first week of puerperium when there is greater risk of thrombo-embolism.
7. Discuss with the cardiologist the question of cardiac surgery and the possible obstetric implications of this.

Congenital heart disease

The general principles for the management of rheumatic heart disease apply also to patients with congenital lesions. Examples of congenital heart lesion encountered in pregnancy are:

1. Patent ductus arteriosus. This causes a permanent arteriovenous shunt. It is diagnosed by the characteristic machinery murmur. Can be trated by ligation during pregnancy if necessary but this operation is usually done before patient becomes pregnant, as most cases are treated in childhood.
2. Coarctation of the aorta. Suspected when blood pressure is higher in arms than legs. Danger of rupture of aorta and cerebral haemorrhage. Patients may require prolonged hospitalisation and need very careful assessment in deciding manner of delivery.
3. Atrial septal defect gives a left to right heart shunt. Medical treatment should be employed during pregnancy and patients with uncomplicated left to right shunts usually do well. The defect should be closed at a suitable time after delivery.

4. Ventricular septal defect causes left to right heart shunt. If reversal of shunt occurs it causes congestive failure. Eisenmenger's syndrome consists of ventricular septal defect with right ventricular hypertrophy, dextrorotation of the aorta and pulmonary hypertension. It is the most dangerous form of congenital heart disease in pregnancy and the maternal mortality may be as high as 40 per cent.
5. Fallot's Tetralogy. In these cases pulmonary artery stenosis is present with ventricular septal defect, right to left shunting and an over-riding aorta. Pregnancy is best avoided but can be supervised on general medical principles.

Cardiomyopathies
These are being increasingly recognised.

1. Hypertrophic obstructive cardiomyopathy, often familial. There is asymmetrical hypertrophy of the ventricles causing obstruction of valves. Increased blood volume during pregnancy may temporarily reduce obstruction. β-blockers are used in treatment.
2. Puerperal cardiomyopathy. This degenerative condition of heart muscle seems to be liable to occur in African patients and is sometimes fatal. It may present as sudden left ventricular failure shortly after delivery.

Maternal mortality
Although the number of deaths from heart disease associated with pregnancy is declining, the proportion of all maternal deaths due to heart disease is increasing. The mortality rate from heart disease associated with pregnancy in recent years is around 0·5 per cent. It is increased according to the severity of the disease and the degree of antenatal care given to the patient.

Heart disease accounts for about 10 per cent of maternal deaths. Avoidable factors have been found to be present in many cases; this emphasises the importance of early diagnosis and adequate treatment.

Perinatal mortality
Both premature labour and intrauterine growth retardation have been reported in association with cardiac disease but generally perinatal mortality is not increased.

Conclusion
With good supervision, the patient with heart disease should

survive pregnancy without any permanent deterioration in her heart condition. Best results are obtained where the obstetrician and cardiologist work as a team. The obstetrician should be aware of the principles of management of heart disease and the cardiologist should have experience of the problems of pregnancy, labour and delivery. Both specialists should combine to advise the patient regarding the prospects of further pregnancies.

DIABETES IN PREGNANCY

Diabetes mellitus is a chronic familial disease characterised by hyperglycaemia and glycosuria. It is caused by an absolute or relative lack of insulin. There is a slow gradation from normal carbohydrate metabolism to clinical diabetes. In pregnancy, all stages of diabetes give rise to increased maternal and fetal risk. The incidence of clinical diabetes in pregnancy is about 1 in 350.

Classification of diabetes

1. *Pre-diabetes.* Glucose tolerance is normal but the patient has a family history of diabetes or a history of previous big babies (more than 4000 G) or unexplained perinatal deaths. A woman who has a baby of 4500 G has a 50 per cent chance of developing diabetes at some time in her life.
2. *Latent chemical diabetes.* Here an abnormality of glucose tolerance is revealed after administration of steroids. Stress such as pregnancy or infection may also cause abnormal glucose tolerance 'Gestational Diabetes' is a form of latent diabetes which appears during pregnancy and remits after delivery.
3. *Chemical diabetes.* There is an abnormal response to a glucose load without stress but the fasting blood sugar (FBS) remains normal.
4. *Clinical diabetes* generally presents with typical symptoms (polydipsia, polyuria etc.). Both fasting blood sugars (FBS) and random blood sugars (RBS) are abnormal and response to glucose load is definitely abnormal.

Effect of pregnancy on diabetes
Pregnancy is diabetogenic.

1. Diabetes in later life is much more common in multiparae than in nulliparae and the incidence appears to increase with the number of pregnancies the patient has had.

2. There is an increase in the insulin requirement from the 16th week of pregnancy onwards. The fall in the renal threshold which occurs at this time may result in a heavy loss of glucose in the urine and consequent gluconeogenesis and ketosis.

Effect of diabetes on pregnancy

There is increased fetal loss mainly due to intauterine death during the last 6 weeks of pregnancy. Premature delivery is therefore indicated and 37 weeks is the time most favoured. At that stage, neonatal complications, particularly respiratory distress syndrome are less common.

The cause of intrauterine death in diabetes is obscure. Post mortem examination of the fetus usually shows hypertrophy of the β-cell islets in the pancreas. This is a response to maternal hyperglycaemia and may lead in turn to hypoglycaemia in the fetus and neonate.

The perinatal loss in diabetes is around 10 per cent although figures as low as 3 per cent have been reported.

Diagnosis of diabetes in pregnancy

Investigation of glycosuria

At every antenatal attendance the urine should be tested with 'Clinistix' which is specific for glucose. Glycosuria occurs in about 9 per cent of normal pregnant women and is usually due to a low renal threshold for glucose.

If glycosuria is present once before 16 weeks gestation or on two occasions after 16 weeks a glucose tolerance test should be done. In the first instance a modified test is done as follows. After blood has been taken for FBS the patient is given a drink of 50 G glucose in 300 ml water: the second blood sugar specimen is taken 2 hours later. If this is more than 120 mg per 100 ml (6 mmol/L) or 20 mg (1 mmol/L) above the fasting level a standard oral glucose tolerance test is required.

The oral glucose tolerance test is generally preferred to the intravenous test. Although the latter is more sensitive it is inconvenient and frequent samples are necessary. The oral test is considered to be more physiological.

The upper limits of normal on an oral glucose tolerance test are:

Fasting: 100 mg/100 ml (5 mmol/L)
1 hour: 160 mg/100 ml (8 mmol/L)
2 hours: 120 mg/100 ml (6 mmol/L)

Indications for glucose tolerance testing in pregnancy

1. Glycosuria – as described above.
2. Family history of diabetes.
3. Previous baby more than 4000 G.
4. Previous unexplained perinatal death(s).
5. Hydramnios.
6. Obesity or excessive weight gain in present pregnancy.

The first diagnosis of diabetes is made during pregnancy in 35 per cent of cases.

Complications of diabetes in pregnancy

1. Urinary tract infection is increased. All patients should be screened for asymptomatic bacteruria.
2. Monilial vulvo-vaginitis may be troublesome.
3. Pre-eclampsia is more common in diabetes but the true incidence may be difficult to find (hypertension greater than 140/90 mmHg is found in 25 per cent diabetics in early pregnancy. Proteinuria may be due to diabetic nephropathy and oedema may be partly a pressure effect).
4. Hydramnios is found in a large proportion of diabetics about the 30th week, but should have decreased by 37 weeks in properly managed patients. There is no satisfactory explanation for the cause of hydramnios in most cases: it may merely be associated with a big baby and big placenta.

Management of diabetes in pregnancy

1. *Teamwork is essential.* The team consists of:
   a. The patient, without whose co-operation nothing can be achieved.
   b. The obstetrician, who must communicate with the others at all times.
   c. The diabetic specialist (not all physicians are specialists in diabetes and not all diabetic specialists have knowledge about the management of diabetes in pregnancy).
   d. The paediatrician.

2. *The principles of treatment* are:
   a. Each patient treated as an individual.
   b. Strict metabolic control.
   c. Adequate time in hospital antenatally.
   d. Monitoring of fetal growth.
   e. Assessment of fetal maturity.

    f. Early, timed delivery.

    g. Intensive neonatal care.

3. *Diet.* Between 150–250 G carbohydrate is allowed. There is no restriction in fat or protein intake unless there is excessive weight gain.

4. *Insulin.* The requirement increases from 16 weeks onwards. Often 2 or 3 doses of soluble insulin are required daily or else 2 doses soluble + isophane insulin.

    The object should be to maintain the FBS around 60 to 80 mg per 100 ml and the RBS less than 120 mg per 100 ml.

    Strict control of blood glucose levels is an essential part of management. Oral hypoglycaemic agents are generally unsuitable for use in pregnancy.

5. *Antenatal hospitalisation.* The patient should be admitted for stabilisation around 24 weeks. This usually takes about a week. She should be readmitted at 32 weeks and stay in hospital until after delivery.

6. *Fetal monitoring.* Every attempt should have been made to assess maturity in early pregnancy. Fetal growth should be studied by serial oestriol excretion measurements and ultrasonic biparietal cephalometry. If the diabetes is kept well controlled, growth of the fetus should not be excessive.

    Before delivery the lecithin-sphingomyelin ratio of the amniotic fluid should be estimated. Anomalous results occur in diabetes and clinical management need not be dictated by this test but it is useful and its wider application is necessary so that results can be properly evaluated.

7. *Preparations for delivery.* All members of the team should be informed of the plan for delivery which generally takes place at 37 weeks.

    On the morning of delivery the patient has no breakfast. A reduced dose of insulin, commonly half the normal dose, is given. Carbohydrate intake is in the form of an intravenous glucose drip. Thereafter, glucose intake and insulin dosage are decided on a 4-hourly basis depending on the results of urine tests for glucose and ketones and on blood sugar estimations.

8. *Delivery.* In most cases induction of labour by amniotomy and oxytocin drip can be employed but there should be an early resort to Caesarean section if there is no progress after 6–8 hours or if some added complication arises.

    General anaesthesia is best avoided and epidural block is preferable for Caesarean section.

9. *Neonatal care.* The large, fat baby of the diabetic mother is

particularly liable to respiratory distress syndrome (it occurs in about 25 per cent). Neonatal hypoglycaemia may occur due to β-cell hyperactivity. Hyperbilirubinaemia can also occur. The importance of early expert paediatric care cannot be overemphasised.

Once the early dangers of respiratory distress, hypoglycaemia and hyperbilirubinaemia have been overcome, the baby's progress is likely to be normal.

10. *Postnatal treatment of mother.* The immediate postpartum insulin requirement is likely to be about half the pre-delivery dose and reduction can be gradual thereafter. Patients with diabetes require intensive care and prolonged hospitalisation during pregnancy. They should give consideration to sterilisation after two or three pregnancies.

6

Maternal mortality

Modern improvements in the maternity services and the general advance of medicine have resulted in a dramatic reduction in the deaths of women due to pregnancy and childbirth, but those deaths which still occur are worth examining in great detail and provide lessons for all engaged in the practice of obstetrics.

In Britain, detailed information on maternal deaths is available through the *Confidential Enquiries into Maternal Deaths*. These enquiries, which assess all available information with great thoroughness, have reviewed maternal deaths in England and Wales since 1952 and in Scotland since 1965. One of the chief features of the investigation is the assessment of any avoidable factors which may have played a part in the ensuing death. The intention of this is to indicate situations where the level of obstetric care fell short of commonly accepted practice. The careful assessment of each death by the doctors concerned and by the regional assessors has made a contribution to the reduction in maternal mortality because it gives an opportunity to consider errors of management or faults in the organisation of the maternity services.

The most recent published report deals with maternal deaths in England and Wales for the three year period 1970–72. In this report a maternal death is defined as one occurring during pregnancy, during labour or as a consequence of pregnancy, within one year of delivery or abortion. Deaths are classified as 'true' maternal deaths if *directly* due to pregnancy and as 'associated' if due to other causes in pregnancy or the puerperium. (The International Federation of Obstetrics and Gynaecology (FIGO) recommends that only deaths occurring within 42 days of delivery or abortion are classified as maternal deaths.)

The 1970–72 Report reviews 590 deaths – 355 true maternal deaths and 251 associated deaths. The maternal mortality rate in this series was 12·9 per 100 000 births. Considerable regional variation was noted e.g. in Oxford the figure was 5·9 and in Leeds 17·2.

Avoidable factors were considered to be present in 191 of the 355 true maternal deaths (53·8 per cent) and in 49 of the 251 associated deaths (19·5 per cent). The avoidable factor was usually a failure to provide appropriate care. During 1972, 90 per cent of all births occurred in NHS hospitals. A change noted in the 1970–72 report was the reduction in the number of births to women with many children. In 1965, 4·0 per cent of deliveries were to mothers having their fifth or later children, whereas in 1972 the proportion had decreased to 1·9 per cent.

The main causes of death were:

1. Abortion.
2. Pulmonary embolism.
3. Toxaemia (i.e. pre-eclampsia and eclampsia).
4. Ectopic pregnancy.
5. Sepsis.

These and some other causes of death are worth some special comment.

Abortion

This remains the largest single cause of maternal death. During 1970–72 deaths from illegal abortion fell while those from legal abortion rose so that the two figures were practically equal.

The most dangerous methods of inducing abortion appeared to be utus paste and laminaria tents. Dilatation and curettage and vacuum aspiration seemed to be the safest, but one death was due to the introduction of positive pressure by the suction curette. Gas embolism in association with vacuum curettage and laparoscopic sterilisation was responsible for two of the 12 deaths from abortion in Scotland in the years 1972 to 1975.

Pulmonary embolism

Second to abortion, this was by far the most frequent cause of death. Many pulmonary emboli occur suddenly and without warning but warning signs of puerperal thrombo-embolism were present in 14 of 30 women delivered vaginally and in 7 of 17 delivered by Caesarean section. These signs may include pleuritic pain which may be treated with antibiotics without its significance being realised.

Amniotic fluid embolism, which is a different entity entirely, is a cause of maternal death which is difficult to prevent.

Aetiological factors in pulmonary thrombo-embolism are:

1. Increasing age.
2. Increasing parity.
3. Operations, such as Caesarean section.
4. Restricted activity – e.g. 'bed rest' for toxaemia.
5. Sickle cell disease (3 of 72 women).
6. Suppression of lactation with oestrogens was a possible factor in 12 of 37 women who died from puerperal thrombo-embolism.

Toxaemia

This includes eclampsia. One or more avoidable factors were present in 66 per cent of all cases of toxaemia and in 76 per cent of those in which fits occurred.

Poor antenatal care remains the most common factor – the patient, general practitioner and consultant all have varied responsibility for this.

Ectopic pregnancy

There were 34 deaths, more than in the report for the previous triennium. 17 patients died at home or in an ambulance and 7 died in hospital while awaiting operation. When the diagnosis of ectopic pregnancy is made, immediate operation is indicated. Resuscitation should not *precede* but should be coincident with operation.

Obviously the only way to reduce deaths from ectopic pregnancy is to have a high 'index of suspicion' and take quick action accordingly.

Sepsis

There were 70 deaths from puerperal sepsis, of which 38 followed abortion, 15 followed vaginal delivery and 17 followed surgical procedures. Avoidable factors were present in 50 of the 70 deaths and attention was drawn to a frequent failure to take specimens for bacteriological examination, particularly in cases of prolonged labour and ruptured membranes.

Haemorrhage

In the report 'haemorrhage' includes abruptio placentae, placenta praevia and postpartum haemorrhage but not abortion, ectopic pregnancy or ruptured uterus.

If abortion and ectopic are included, it appears that haemorrhage was a major factor in 105 of 355 true maternal deaths.

Important points about haemorrhage are:

1. The risk increases with age and parity.

2. The proportion of avoidable factors has remained unchanged (52 per cent).

3. Every case of antepartum haemorrhage requires early admission to hospital and the Flying Squad should, where necessary give blood before transferring the patient.

4. Early and adequate blood transfusion (using Group O Rhesus negative blood if necessary) will help to prevent the complications of abruptio placentae. Transfusion should be monitored by central venous pressure where possible.

5. Caesarean section for placenta praevia should be performed or directly supervised by a consultant. The danger of morbid adhesion of the placenta to the lower segment scar should be remembered.

6. A coagulation disorder should be suspected in all cases of postpartum haemorrhage.

7. Hysterectomy should be performed if bleeding from an atonic uterus cannot be controlled by bimanual compression, compression of the aorta and appropriate drugs.

Caesarean section

There were 111 deaths associated with Caesarean section in England and Wales in 1970–72. The fatality rate was 1 per 1000 Caesarean sections performed in NHS hospitals. The Scottish report for the years 1972–75 suggests that this figure may now be lower.

One or more avoidable factors was present in 51 cases (45·9 per cent). This is a higher proportion than in any series reported since 1952, when avoidable factors were found in only 29·7 per cent.

In Scotland, in the years 1965–71, 26 per cent of maternal deaths were in women delivered by Caesarean section. Many of the women who died were already seriously ill when operation was decided on, but a number of deaths were the direct result of operative complications. The Scottish report comments that, in deciding upon an elective Caesarean section for an indication which is not mandatory, the obstetrician opting for the operation opts also for its risks, which may be minimal, may be acceptable, but are not entirely negligible.

Anaesthesia

The total number of deaths from anaesthesia has fallen, but avoidable factors were present in more than 75 per cent of cases. Most of these involved junior staff, suggesting a need for better supervision by more experienced anaesthetists.

Women suffering from obstetric emergencies are often gravely at risk and deserve the knowledge and skill of an experienced anaesthetist.

The mother at risk
The Scottish Report (1965–71) identifies certain categories of women who are at greater risk of maternal death.

1. Mothers aged more than 35 years.
2. Those of high parity (5 or more).
3. Those of lower social class (especially wives of unskilled workers) and those from overcrowded home conditions.
4. Unmarried mothers.

Conclusion
Although the number of maternal deaths continues to fall, the presence of avoidable factors in about half of the cases leaves no room for complacency.

7

Perinatal mortality and morbidity

Perinatal mortality is defined as the sum of stillbirths and deaths during the first week of life and the perinatal mortality rate is this number expressed per 1000 total births. The main contribution to the study of this subject in the last 20 years was the British Perinatal Mortality Survey of 1958 when there was an intensive study of all singleton births which took place in the week 3–9 March 1958. The report of this survey was published in 1963. A second report in 1969 gave more detailed analysis of some aspects of the survey and, in 1970, there followed another study, the British Births Survey, the result of which was published in 1975. In 1958, the perinatal mortality rate in England and Wales was 35·1 per 1000; in 1969 it was 23 per 1000 and in 1976 was 18 per 1000.

Main causes of perinatal death

1. Malformations
2. Prematurity
3. Asphyxia ± birth trauma

Prematurity is the main cause of neonatal deaths, and nearly half the total perinatal deaths occur before 38 weeks.

Post-mortem findings in perinatal death

In the survey of 1958 the main post-mortem findings were:

Cause of perinatal death	
Intra-partum anoxia	22.9
Congenital malformations	19·0
Antepartum anoxia	11·2
Antepartum fetal death with no lesion	10·9
Cerebral birth trauma ± intrapartum asphyxia	10·0
Hyaline membrane ± intra- ventricular haemorrhage	9·6
Pneumonia	4·8
Rhesus Iso-immunisation	4·3

Anoxia was therefore the commonest cause of perinatal death and the combination of intrapartum anoxia and/or birth trauma caused almost one third of the total deaths.

Factors influencing perinatal mortality

Social, environmental and obstetrical factors are all important.

1. *Geographical.* Perinatal mortality is higher in the North and West of Britain and lower in the South and East.
2. Age of mother. Women over 30 years have a progressively increasing risk of perinatal death. Best results are in women aged 20–24.
3. *Parity.* Second babies have the best chance of survival. First babies have more than the average risk of death and fourth and subsequent babies are most at risk.
4. *Social class.* Perinatal mortality doubles from social class 1 to social class 5.
5. *Past obstetric history.* A history of previous abortions, perinatal deaths and/or premature delivery increases the risk.
6. *Antenatal care and place of delivery.* Best results occur in women who have high quality antenatal care and are delivered in specialist units. Women who are never seen by obstetric specialists and those booking late or transferred late for confinement in hospital have an increased risk.
7. *Gestational age and birth weight* are immensely important factors. Babies are most safely born between 38 and 42 weeks. More than half of the total perinatal deaths occur in babies weighing less than 2500 g. In the survey of 1958 it was reported that one third of these babies were born at 38 weeks or later: this emphasised the importance of the 'small for dates' baby.
8. *Toxaemia.* Pre-eclampsia and related conditions increase the risk, which rises with the severity of the toxaemia, being specially marked when proteinuria is present.
9. *Bleeding.* All types of bleeding during pregnancy increase risk to the fetus. Bleeding before 28 weeks increases the risk even when the pregnancy continues to term. Both placenta praevia and abruptio placentae increase the risk as does antepartum haemorrhage of uncertain origin, particularly if associated with prematurity.
10. *Labour and delivery.* Both long (>24 hours) and short labours are associated with a greater risk to the baby.
    Breech delivery is associated with increased risk especially if the baby is smaller or larger than average. Breech delivery

appears to be more dangerous in the multipara than in the primigravida.

Forceps delivery carries an increased mortality when the baby weighs more than 4000 g.

Perinatal deaths after Caesarean section are related to the indication for the section, although there seems to be an increased risk of hyaline membrane disease in these cases.

Lessons from the study of perinatal mortality

It is quite clear that perinatal mortality is related to the quality of maternity services. Important points to be remembered are:

1. There must be careful selection of high risk patients who should be confined in suitable units. Even where hospital confinement is almost universal, not all hospitals offer every type of monitoring facility and many maternity hospitals have no direct link with a neonatal paediatric department.

2. Knowledge of gestational age is of prime importance. This information can best be obtained if the woman attends for antenatal care as early as possible. Women who present later for antenatal care are at increased risk.

3. Use all available antenatal tests (e.g. sonar, urinary oestriols, amniotic lecithin/sphingomyelin ratio) and interpret them intelligently.

4. Recognise the value and dangers of induction, accelerated and augmented labour, and intrapartum fetal monitoring. Again, intelligent use and interpretation is necessary.

5. Recognise and treat toxaemia as early as possible.

6. Remember the risk of vaginal bleeding at all stages in pregnancy.

7. Remember the dangers of difficult forceps and breech deliveries.

8. Remember the importance of social and environmental factors and where necessary enlist the help of social workers and others.

As has already been stated the major causes of perinatal death are congenital malformations, prematurity and asphyxia ± birth trauma.

Malformations cannot in general be prevented but many may be diagnosed by amniocentesis and the woman can be offered termination.

Premature labour is difficult to prevent but an attempt should be made to do so (e.g. by cervical suture in cases of cervical incompetence, by admission of appropriate cases to hospital for rest) and some cases can be treated with drugs (e.g. salbutamol, ritodrine).

Unnecessarily early induction of labour ('iatrogenic prematurity') should be avoided.

Asphyxia and/or birth trauma can be treated by recognising antenatal fetal growth retardation, by careful intrapartum monitoring and by the skill and experience of those responsible for the woman's care in labour.

Finally, the neonatal death rate has been and can be greatly reduced by the extension and development of paediatric services.

Every perinatal death should be the subject of an enquiry at a local perinatal mortality meeting and data should be available for national assessment also.

Perinatal morbidity

The quality of life of surviving infants is very difficult to assess because of the lack of reliable data. The effect of congenital malformations varies according to their type and severity. Brain damage following birth trauma still occurs but has become unusual. Babies born before 33 weeks have an increased risk of mental handicap but this may be reduced by intensive neonatal care.

Mental development may also be retarded or abnormal in cases of fetal growth retardation but treatment of such complications as neonatal hypoglycaemia may have reduced the risk. The adverse effect of smoking during pregnancy on fetal growth and development has stimulated publicity in the attempt to reduce this habit.

Mothers of high parity and low social class are more likely to have children who are 'born to fail'. Every attempt should be made to get such mothers to take advantage of the available obstetric and paediatric services.

Part II Gynaecology

8

History and examination of the gynaecological patient

HISTORY

This may be the most important part of the gynaecological consultation, and should always be taken with care. On some occasions the whole diagnosis may be revealed by the history, if the doctor is prepared to listen, although in other instances the patient's account of her symptoms may be almost irrelevant and treatment will be directed towards the physical signs elicited on examination – e.g. in the case of a large symptomless abdominal tumour.

The following facts should be elicited in all cases:

1. *History of present complaint.*
This should be written down briefly in simple words. Cumbrous terms of Greek or Latin origin are best avoided – e.g. it is better to write 'frequent heavy periods' rather than 'epimenorrhagia'.

It should be remembered that the patient's stated complaint may on occasion mask her real problem. This applies no matter whether the complaint is physical or psychological, e.g. vaginal discharge may really be due to sexual dissatisfaction while alleged sexual problems (which it is now fashionable to discuss) may be due to marital disharmony which has its basis in financial difficulties.

2. *Previous medical history*
A brief record should be made of any serious illness or of any surgical operation, particular attention being paid to abdominal operations or any gynaecological procedures.

3. *Obstetric history*
This should also be recorded briefly, with the ages of children and the nature of the deliveries (spontaneous, forceps, Caesarean section etc).

4. *Menstrual history*

This requires to be recorded in some detail, including

a. Age at menarche.

b. Menstrual cycle recorded as a figure e.g. 4/28 making sure the patient understands that the first day of bleeding is the first day of menstruation.

c. Amount of menstrual loss is bound to be a subjective impression but some idea of amount can be obtained by asking the number of towels used and whether clots are passed.

d. Date of last menstrual period.

5. *Marital and sexual history*

This can be taken at this point, as the previous enquiries, conducted in an objective manner, will probably have put the patient at her ease sufficiently to give a clear and relevant account. The gynaecologist owes it to his patient to discuss sexual matters with a combination of gentleness, frankness and dignity.

Taking an adequate gynaecological history is an art and part of the art is to conduct the interview expeditiously while allowing enough time for the patient to talk.

EXAMINATION

1. *General*

The examination should be conducted in privacy with the assistance of a nurse. Few gynaecologists have the time or inclination to conduct a detailed general medical examination but the opportunity should be taken to observe the patient's general appearance and answer the question 'Does she look well or ill?' A comment can also be made regarding her mental and psychological attitude although written remarks about this on an outpatient casesheet should be brief and objective. Systemic examination can be done as indicated by the history (e.g. examination of the heart and lungs in someone with a history of cough or dyspnoea) and appropriate investigations such as X-rays or electrocardiographs ordered.

Blood should be sent for haemoglobin estimation.

2. *Examination of the breasts*

This should be a routine part of gynaecological examination and is best done with the patient sitting up, each quadrant of the breast and also the axillae being palpated in a methodical manner.

3. *Abdominal examination*

After inspection of scars and any visible lump, the examiner, standing on the patient's right, can best palpate her upper abdomen, including liver and spleen, with his right hand; the lower abdomen, including any masses arising from the pelvis, is best palpated with the left hand, feeling for the upper edge of any pelvic tumour with the ulnar border of the hand.

4. *Vaginal examination*

This is usually made in either the dorsal or left lateral position. Clear instructions should be given to the patient so that she is co-operative and relaxed.

Dorsal position. The patient, lying on her back, is asked to bend her knees up, put her heels together and then separate her knees wide apart. An additional useful instruction is for her to have the soles of her feet touching each other – to do this she must abduct her thighs fully.

Left lateral position. The patient is asked to lie on her side, bring her bottom to the edge of the couch, keep the left leg almost straight and flex the right leg fully at hip and knee.

Inspection of external genitals. This is the first part of the examination, note being made of evidence of vulvitis, Bartholinitis, warts etc. The patient is asked to cough or bear down to reveal any utero-vaginal prolapse.

Speculum examination. Passage of the speculum should be gentle, painless and expeditious. Nothing is more likely to lose the patient's confidence than fussiness, coarseness or ineptitude in this part of the examination. It is the usual practice to lubricate the speculum with either water or a little clear sterile jelly so that bacteriological or cytological specimens are not spoiled by antiseptics or creams. Speculum examination should precede digital vaginal examination although some gynaecologists (the author among them) prefer to locate the cervix first by gentle palpation with one finger. This provides a guide for the direction along which the speculum should be introduced.

For examination in the dorsal position, Cusco's bivalve speculum is a popular instrument, whereas for the lateral position Sims' speculum is best. The lateral position is very useful for assessing descent of the anterior vaginal wall and for viewing the cervix when the uterus is retroverted.

Cervical smear. Before taking the smear, the appearance of the cervix should be noted. The smear can be taken with an Ayre's spatula or similar instrument or with a small piece of rough dry sponge, which will provide not only a specimen for cytology but also a 'sponge biopsy' for histology.

Bimanual examination of the uterus and adnexa. The examiner should note and record in a systematic manner the following facts about the uterus:

1. Size
2. Shape
3. Position
4. Mobility
5. Consistency

Adnexal swellings should also be described as accurately as possible, noting their size, consistency, mobility and attachment to the uterus.

Special diagnostic techniques. These should be used as indicated. They include:

1. Ultrasonography for many indications.
2. Colposcopy where there is suspicion of cervical carcinoma.
3. Hysterography for infertility or diagnosis of Mullerian duct anomalies.
4. Laparoscopy for many indications.

The patient's reaction to vaginal examination may give an indication of her psychosexual attitude but apart from obvious cases of vaginismus or women who complain of offensive vaginal discharge which can neither be seen nor smelled there is usually little to record.

The art of gynaecological history-taking and examination cannot be learned from books but only by practical demonstration and experience. The basic principles which are to be put into practice include:

1. Sympathy
2. Objectivity
3. Confidentiality
4. Gentleness
5. Efficiency

Careful, systematic recording of results is essential, both for efficiency and for medico-legal reasons. Finally, remember that fear of serious organic abnormality or disease (usually cancer) is still probably the commonest reason for attendance as a gynaecological outpatient. The most powerful therapy is often reassurance. When the gynaecologist says 'I have examined you and find nothing wrong' he may have cured his patient.

9

Menstrual disorders

AMENORRHEA

Primary amenorrhea
Amenorrhea is a symptom, not a disease, and may have many causes. Menstruation commonly begins between the ages of 10 and 16 years. Primary amenorrhea is not usually investigated before the age of 18 years. Girls who have not menstruated at what is thought by them or their mothers to be the normal age are sometimes referred to the gynaecologist. Examination and reassurance may be all that is required if normality is confirmed. Primary amenorrhea should not be thought of as a symptom on its own but in association with the other signs of secondary sexual development, which may be normal or abnormal.

Primary amenorrhea with normal secondary sexual development
1. Anatomical causes such as imperforate hymen causing cryptomenorrhea and absence of uterus in a genetically normal female.
2. Testicular feminisation syndrome (Androgen insensitivity). In this syndrome, a normal male karyotype (46 × 7) is associated with an apparently normal female figure and temperament. Clinical features include:

   a. Good breast development.
   b. Absent or scanty sexual hair.
   c. Normal or hypoplastic vulva.
   d. Short blind vagina.
   e. Absent uterus.
   f. Intra-abdominal, inguinal or labial testes.

The testes appear to produce testosterone in normal male amounts, and also oestrogens. Insensitivity to androgens seems to be the cause of the syndrome as masculinisation does not occur in the presence of normal androgen levels.

Diagnosis is based on the clinical features, the finding of a normal male karotype on chromosome analysis and plasma testosterone levels well above the female range.

Treatment. Gonadectomy is recommended to avoid the risk of malignancy which is of the order of 5 per cent.

Postoperatively, replacement oestrogen therapy is indicated to avoid menopausal-type symptoms.

Patients with this condition should be handled with kindness and care. The information that an apparently normal attractive girl will never have children and will require an operation to have her 'ovaries' removed can be devastating.

Primary amenorrhea with clinical signs of masculinisation
Buccal smear and chromosome analysis are necessary in all cases before a diagnosis can be made.
1. Gonadal dysgenesis with a Y chromosome present.
   As stated above, gonadectomy is necessary, both to avoid malignancy and to arrest the masculinising changes produced by functioning testicular tissue.
2. Congenital adrenal hyperplasia. If the patient has a chromatin positive smear and a 46 XX karyotype the signs of masculinisation (particularly clitoral enlargement) are due to excessive androgen production. Excessive production of androgens by the adrenals can be suppressed by the administration of cortisone.

Secondary amenorrhea
The commonest cause of secondary amenorrhea is, of course, pregnancy and the possibility of this should always be considered, even in the most unlikely cases, such as those patients who have been attending for a long time with oligomenorrhea and amenorrhea from other causes.

Functional disorders of the hypothalamic pituitary unit.
Emotional stress. This may inhibit the production of hypothalamic releasing factors which allow the production of FSH and LH. Secondary amenorrhea is a common complaint among young women in their late teens and early twenties, particularly students, nurses and those starting professional life. Such girls may be living away from home for the first time and numerous emotional factors may be involved. In these cases, abnormality is seldom found and the patient can usually be told that amenorrhea will cause her no harm and menstruation will probably return to normal without treatment.

It is inadvisable and unnecessary to embark on complicated endocrinological investigations and potentially dangerous surgical diagnostic procedures on young healthy women with no evidence of organic disease, who are not complaining of infertility and who are very busy with their studies or careers.

Malnutrition. This may also result in hypothalamic pituitary suppression and lead to secondary amenorrhea. Amenorrhea is common when women are living in conditions of famine. If severe malnutrition occurs at or just before puberty, infertility may be a problem later. An incidence of 75 per cent infertility was reported from concentration camp victims in the Second World War. In modern western society where food is abundant the commonest cause of this type of amenorrhea is anorexia nervosa a disease occurring mostly in adolescents where physical and psychological factors are both at work and where treatment, including psychotherapy, may be very difficult, particularly as the patient may not acknowledge that she is ill. Anorexia nervosa must always be treated energetically as some patients may not recover.

Obesity. As a cause of amenorrhea obesity is more difficult to explain. In these patients the amenorrhea is probably due to the psychic stress which also causes the obesity. Weight reduction, with a well balanced diet should result in cure.

Organic pituitary disease

Sheehan's syndrome. Necrosis of the anterior lobe of the pituitary following a traumatic delivery associated with post partum haemorrhage was described by Sheehan when he was pathologist to the Glasgow Royal Maternity Hospital. Uterine and vaginal atrophy are followed by weight loss, loss of axillary and pubic hair and cachexia. Gonadotrophin excretion is lowered or absent, protein-bound iodine is low, basal metabolic rate is low and anaemia is a feature.

Replacement therapy is with 25 mg of cortisone acetate or its equivalent, daily, plus oestrogens.

Pituitary tumours. Amenorrhea is a common symptom among women with pituitary tumours. A history of headache and visual disturbance in association with amenorrhea should always rouse suspicion. Diagnostic aids include X-ray of the pituitary fossa, a colour visual field investigation and estimation of pituitary gonadotrophins which will be low.

Amenorrhea and galactorrhea

The syndrome of amenorrhea in association with galactorrhea

(which is the secretion of milk in the absence of an appropriate physiological stimulus) has been known since ancient times. Patients with these symptoms are often found to have elevated serum prolactin and reduced serum LH and FSH levels. Hyperprolactinaemia inhibits steroidogenesis in the ovary. Prolactin is a 'stress hormone' and its concentration in the blood may rise after physical or emotional stress. This should be remembered when assessing women with menstrual disturbances.

The response of the breasts to elevated serum prolactin is variable but if the concentration of prolactin is more than 50 ng/ml, galactorrhea is usually present.

Some cases of amenorrhea and galactorrhea may be due to a pituitary adenoma. If there is any radiological abnormality of the pituitary fossa, however minor, a full investigation is indicated: this may involve air-encephalography. Galactorrhea may occur spontaneously or in response to drugs, particularly oestrogens (including oral contraceptives) and dopamine depleting agents such as methyldopa.

In the absence of a pituitary tumour, patients with amenorrhea and galactorrhea may be treated with Bromocriptine, a semi-synthetic ergot alkaloid which acts on the pituitary to suppress prolactin secretion. The usual dose is 2·5 mg two or three times daily. While on treatment with this drug, the patient should use mechanical methods of contraception because there is a risk of pituitary expansion during pregnancy which may lead to compression of the optic chiasma.

Bromocriptine may also be used to suppress puerperal lactation. It does not affect the blood clotting system and there is no evidence that it causes hyperplasia or cancer of the endometrium.

'Post-pill' amenorrhea

Oral contraceptives have been described as the most common iatrogenic cause of amenorrhea. They act by inhibiting gonadotrophin releasing hormone and in some individuals, prolonged hypothalamic suppression can result. There is no way of predicting cases in which it will occur, but women with a previous history of oligomenorrhea and those who have been taking oral contraceptives for a long time may be more liable to develop amenorrhea when the pill is stopped. Recent investigations have cast some doubt on the association between oral contraceptives and subsequent amenorrhea and have emphasised the importance of previous episodes of amenorrhea before oral contraceptive treatment. Whatever the cause, menstruation usually returns to normal spontaneously and the first line of treatment should be to reassure the women about this. If she is anxious about infertility or if amenorrhea persists for as long as a year, treatment with clomiphene is indicated and is usually effective, but the possibility of other causes for the amenorrhea, such as pituitary tumour and primary ovarian failure should always be borne in mind.

Stein–Leventhal syndrome
Amenorrhea or oligomenorrhea is a frequent feature of this syndrome, in which bilateral polycystic ovaries are associated with infertility, hirsutism and menstrual irregularities. Each ovary may be about the size of the uterus, and contains multiple small cysts which have a thin lining of granulosa and a marked luteinisation of the theca interna. The diagnosis should not be made unless both ovaries are shown convincingly to be enlarged: laparoscopy may demonstrate this but sonar with modern grey-scale technique now offers a non-invasive method of visualising and measuring the ovaries and can be used not only to make the diagnosis but to assess the response to treatment.

Examination of the urine shows evidence of excessive gonadotrophin production with a predominance of LH over FSH. Oestrogen excretion is above normal in some patients whereas in those with hirsutism 17-ketosteroid excretion is raised, indicating excessive androgen secretion. The diagnosis may sometimes lack precision because of paradoxical findings and the pathogenesis of the syndrome is obscure. Similarly, the reason for the cure usually brought about by bilateral wedge resection of the ovaries is not clear. The operation probably results somehow in an alteration of the FSH/LH ratio in favour of FSH. Ovarian surgery makes no difference to the hirsutism which is often the patient's primary complaint and it is doubtful whether an otherwise healthy young woman should have an operation unless she is complaining of infertility.

Ovarian tumours
Functioning ovarian tumours may produce both feminising and masculinising effects in varying degrees.

The commonest masculinising tumour is the arrhenoblastoma which first presents clinically with a stage of defeminisation, indicated by amenorrhoea and atrophy of the breasts. A stage of masculinisation with hirsutism, hoarse voice and clitoral hypertrophy follows.

Removal of the tumour results in the return of menstruation

although the signs of masculinisation such as hirsutism may be slow to disappear.

Most arrhenoblastomas occur in women under 30 years of age.

Metabolic diseases

Thyroid. Amenorrhea may be associated with both hypothyroidism and hyperthyroidism. Thyroid function tests should be performed where there is clinical suspicion of dysfunction and appropriate therapy will then probably restore normal menstruation.

Amenorrhea is not the only menstrual disturbance associated with thyroid disease and some patients may present with a complaint of irregular or excessive menstrual bleeding.

Diabetes Mellitus. This is similarly associated with menstrual disturbances and sometimes amenorrhea may be a feature. The well controlled diabetic usually has normal menstruation.

Adrenal disorder. The adrenogenital syndrome usually presents with primary amenorrhea but sometimes virilization may occur after puberty. The disease is caused by an enzyme deficiency which prevents the adrenal from synthesising cortisol and the treatment is cortisone replacement.

Amenorrhea is also a characteristic of Cushing's syndrome where there is hyperfunction of the whole adrenal cortex. Some cases are associated with pituitary tumours (basophil adenomata) as originally described by Cushing, but in others there is adrenal hyperplasia without any pituitary lesion. Urinary and blood corticoids are elevated and cannot be suppressed by cortisone. Amenorrhea is an early symptom of adrenal tumours, in which cases there is an elevation of dehydroisoandrosterone.

DYSMENORRHEA

Dysmenorrhea or menstrual pain is one of the most common disorders in gynaecology and is one of the most important causes of loss of working time among women. It should be remembered that dysmenorrhea is a *symptom*, not a precise pathological process and that each patient who presents with this symptom requires individual consideration.

Primary (or spasmodic) dysmenorrhea

The use of the word 'primary' might suggest that this pain begins with the menarche but this is not usually so. Primary dysmenorrhea is a disorder of ovulating women and the first periods after the menarche are usually painless because they are anovular. As soon as ovulation is established, menstrual pain may begin. Pain usually starts with the onset of bleeding and lasts for a few hours. It is most frequently spasmodic or colicky in nature, situated in the lower abdomen and may be accompanied by diarrhoea, nausea and vomiting.

Factors in the causation of dysmenorrhea

Hormonal. As dysmenorrhea is associated with ovulatory cycles, it seems reasonable to assume that progesterone plays a part in its causation. Under the influence of progesterone, the secretory endometrium synthesises prostaglandin F2α, a hormone which causes contraction of smooth muscles. (When given therapeutically, prostaglandin F2α not only produces uterine contractions but also acts on the gut, giving diarrhoea.)

The spasmodic pain of dysmenorrhea is probably caused by uterine contractions due to the overaction of prostaglandin on the myometrium.

Anatomical. The traditional teaching that spasmodic dysmenorrhea was caused by hypoplasia of the uterus, acute anteversion or retroversion, or stenosis of the cervix has become discredited.

Although anatomical factors may play a part in some cases they are certainly not the main causes.

Psychogenic. Girls complaining of dysmenorrhea are often accompanied by mothers who are all too ready to give a vivid account of the agonies they themselves suffered with menstruation and who may have narrow or distorted ideas about sexual function in general. With the advance of sexual education, spasmodic dysmenorrhea seems to be decreasing, at least in hospital practice.

The management of primary dysmenorrhea begins with a simple explanation to the girl that period pains are not symptoms of disease but of normal female function. This reassurance is backed up by a physical examination after which the gynaecologist can state firmly that he has found no abnormality of the pelvic organs. Further treatment can then be discussed. If the pain is relieved reasonably adequately by simple analgesics such as paracetamol, the girl is told to continue with these. She is also advised to continue normal work and activity during menstruation. If the pain is not relieved by analgesics and interferes considerably with the girl's life and work, a contraceptive pill should be prescribed. This, by suppressing ovulation, converts painful menstruation into painless withdrawal bleeding in most cases. The action of the pill should be described clearly to the patient. She should take this treatment for 6 months, after which she can try the effect of stopping treatment. In many cases a spontaneous cure will have taken place.

If the patient does not wish to have ovulation suppressed a progestational preparation such as dydrogesterone ('Duphaston') 10 mg twice daily, can be given from the fifth to the 25th day of the cycle.

All consultations should take place in private between the patient and the gynaecologist. The mother can be suitably informed and reassured after the discussion.

If relief is not obtained by hormone treatment the question of carrying out a full gynaecological investigation including such measures as pelvic examination under anaesthesia, dilation and curettage or laparoscopy should be decided. Such procedures should not be undertaken lightly in young nulliparous women. The adverse effect of forcible cervical dilatation (once the most popular treatment for dysmenorrhea) upon subsequent pregnancies is well known and laparoscopy also has its own hazards.

Some gynaecologists are still prepared to perform presacral neurectomy for intractable dysmenorrhea and success is occasionally reported, but patients who reach the stage of requiring such an operation may have deeply rooted psychogenic causes which should have been explored by methods other than the use of surgical instruments.

Secondary (or congestive) dysmenorrhea

This is a symptom which generally occurs in the later half of reproductive life and it is usually due to organic disease of the pelvic organs.

The pain of secondary dysmenorrhea usually starts before the menstrual flow and premenstrual tension may be marked. Pain commonly continues through the period but gradually lessens. Dyspareunia is often an associated symptom.

Causes

Endometriosis. The patient with endometriosis is often nulliparous or else a number of years have passed since her last pregnancy. On examination tenderness or irregularity is found in the region of the uterosacral ligaments and there may be additional signs associated with the formation of chocolate cysts of the ovary or with extensive adhesions in the pelvis. Laparoscopy is often indicated to clinch the diagnosis but patients with a substantial pelvic mass will of course require laparotomy for diagnosis and treatment. Ultrasonography does not reveal any features which differentiate endometriosis from other conditions with similar physical signs.

If the signs of endometriosis are doubtful it may be worth carrying out a therapeutic test with dydrogesterone ('Duphaston') 10 mg daily from the fifth to the 25th day of the cycle. This and similar hormone preparations may be used in an attempt at medical treatment. A recent popular treatment is danazol, which apparently interferes with the release of pituitary gonadotrophins and which is given in doses of 200 to 800 mg daily.

Fibroids. These also are commonest in nulliparous or relatively infertile women. The typical fibroid associated with dysmenorrhea is the submucous which protrudes into the uterine cavity and may become a fibroid polyp. During menstruation it causes colicky pains like labour. Menstrual loss is likely to be heavy with clots. If such a fibroid is not obvious on clinical examination, it may be revealed by an ultrasonogram or X-ray hysterogram. The treatment is surgical-myomectomy or hysterectomy as appropriate to the age and parity of the patient and her wishes about further reproduction. Fibroids are a relatively uncommon cause of dysmenorrhea.

Pelvic inflammatory disease. The history of the onset of dysmenorrhea may suggest that it is associated with infection after childbirth or abortion. If clinical examination reveals signs of pelvic inflammatory disease treatment with antibiotics is probably worthwhile in the first instance. If the condition is a chronic one with recurring exacerbations short wave diathermy may be helpful but the patient may eventually have to face the necessity of surgery. Surgery for pelvic inflammatory disease, to be successful, usually requires to be radical, in the form of total hysterectomy and bilateral salpingo-oophorectomy. The possibility of tuberculosis as a cause of pelvic imflammatory disease should be remembered although it is increasingly rare in the western world. The diagnosis should preferably be made by endometrial biopsy and culture before laparotomy so that any operation can be performed under full antituberculous chemotherapy. Pelvic inflammatory disease (with the exception of tuberculosis) is an important cause of dysmenorrhea in parous and sexually active women. Precision in diagnosis may be difficult or impossible but treatment on the general lines suggested above is often effective.

DYSFUNCTIONAL UTERINE BLEEDING

Abnormal uterine bleeding may be associated with lesions of the genital tract which are clearly identifiable, for example, carcinoma of cervix or endometrium, retained products of conception, fibroids or ovarian tumours. Dysfunctional uterine bleeding is abnormal bleeding which is not associated with neoplasms, pregnancy, inflammation, blood dyscrasia, trauma or hormone administration. The diagnosis of dysfunctional bleeding should not be made unless these other common organic conditions have been excluded. In most cases this means that the patient has a careful bimanual examination, a cervical smear and a diagnostic curettage performed before the diagnosis is made and treatment started. Some patients will also require estimation of hormone levels and investigations such as ultrasonography, hysterography or laparoscopy to give a more detailed picture of the function and form of the uterus and ovaries. In every case the gynaecologist should consider the possibility that the bleeding may be a manifestation of a general medical disease (such as hypothyroidism) or a psychogenic cause (such as marital disharmony).

There have been numerous hypotheses on the cause of dysfunctional bleeding. There have also been numerous classifications. A simple and practical one is to divide the cases into those associated with failure of ovulation and those in which ovulation takes place and the endometrium develops a secretory pattern.

Anovulatory bleeding
Most cases (perhaps 80 per cent) of dysfunctional uterine bleeding are of this type. *Metropathia haemorrhagica* was the name given by Schröder in 1915 to a disorder produced by abnormal persistence of unruptured ovarian follicles, the absence of corpora lutea and the consequent production of cystic glandular hyperplasia of the endometrium. The fundamental endocrine pathology of these changes remains obscure.

Causes
Central. The cause of the disturbance of ovarian function may be central, in the hypothalamic-pituitary axis, and may be associated with psychogenic or constitutional factors related to the woman's general health. A central cause is also the probable reason for the frequency of anovulatory bleeding at the extremes of reproductive life in the adolescent and in the pre-menopausal woman when the whole endocrine machinery associated with ovulation is running-in or running-down. More than half of the patients who present with dysfunctional bleeding are over 45 years of age and about one fifth are adolescents.

Local. Local causes, in the ovary itself, may be important in the pre-menopausal woman but are not always identifiable. Functioning ovarian tumours may be associated with anovulatory bleeding.

Diagnosis of anovulatory bleeding

The diagnosis of anovulatory bleeding is made definitively by examination of endometrial curettings obtained during the second half of the menstrual cycle. In the adolescent girl, however, curettage is often best avoided unless bleeding is very severe. The length of the cycle may be extremely variable during the first two or three years after the menarche and when bleeding problems arise in the adolescent it may be reasonable to employ hormone therapy without preliminary curettage which is not always an uncomplicated operation in the young nullipara.

A similar period of menstrual variability may occur for several years between the reproductive and menopausal phases but at this time of life the risk of cancer is a substantial one and the gynaecologist should always carry out a full investigation including curettage. Hormone therapy should never be given blindly to perimenopausal women.

The continuous proliferation of the endometrium in cases of anovulatory bleeding is caused by constant unopposed oestrogen stimulation and not by excessive output of oestrogens. The endometrial histology may vary from a slightly exaggerated proliferation to marked cystic glandular hyperplasia.

The clinical history in the classic case of metropathia haemorrhagica is that of amenorrhea for about 6 weeks followed by prolonged and profuse bleeding but all kinds of variations occur.

The gynaecologist must take a careful history, enquiring about variations in the woman's normal menstrual pattern, about ovulatory symptoms such as inter-menstrual pain, pre-menstrual tension and dysmenorrhea, about menopausal symptoms like hot flushes, sweats and headaches, about any medication she has been taking and about the possibility of pregnancy, for after all, the commonest cause of bleeding after amenorrhea is not anovulation but abortion.

Treatment of anovulatory bleeding

The treatment of anovulatory bleeding should have as its first aim the transformation of proliferative into secretory endometrium and thus the restoration of normal menstruation.

Medical. The ideal medical treatment is a combination of oestrogen and progesterone as found in most contraceptive pills. These, given in a dose of four tablets daily for four or five days will gener-ally be successful in stopping bleeding. The treatment can then be continued as one tablet daily for the remainder of the usual three week dosage regime. After three or four months, treatment should be stopped in the hope that menstruation will return to normal, which it often does spontaneously. A similar regime may be employed with a pure progestational agent such as Norethisterone (Norethuterone) or medroxyprogesterone acetate.

Surgical. The rôle of uterine curettage in the diagnosis of anovulatory bleeding has already been mentioned. Curettage also is a form of surgical treatment and before the advent of hormone therapy it was the usual initial treatment. It was claimed that thorough curettage by removing the basal layer of the endo-metrium, stimulated regrowth in a more normal pattern and it was said that almost half the cases of anovulatory bleeding could be controlled in this way. Such a view is almost certainly an over-simplification but there is no doubt that many women's symptoms will improve after curettage alone. Hysterectomy is of course the ultimate solution to the problem of dysfunctional uterine bleeding. The gynaecologist's difficulty is knowing when to recommend it. Hysterectomy may be the treatment of choice for the older woman who has completed her family and such patients often welcome the prospect of definitive surgery rather than long term hormone treatment. As with any patient for whom hysterectomy is proposed, the gynaecologist must explain the nature and results of the opera-tion in understandable terms, paying particular attention to questions about sexual or menopausal problems. When a woman is averse to hysterectomy it is rarely advisable to apply strong per-suasion to make her change her mind. In a younger woman for whom reproductive function is important, a trial of oestrogen/pro-gesterone therapy (as described above) may be given and this should be followed by cyclic progestational therapy. These treatments are not a cure. They merely provide a form of hormonal homeostasis and allow spontaneous cure to take place after the treatment is stopped.

Ovulatory bleeding
Dysfunctional uterine bleeding is associated with a secretory pattern of endometrium and is more difficult to treat with hor-mones than is anovulatory bleeding.

Cause of ovulatory bleeding
Bleeding associated with secretory endometrium should be re-

garded as anatomical until proved otherwise. Some of the most serious cases of menstrual bleeding I have seen have been associated with a small submucous fibroid which has escaped detection at first examination and curettage. If all anatomical factors can be excluded the bleeding is assumed to be due to some abnormality of ovarian function, such as:

1. Defects in follicular maturation with an inadequate luteal phase.
2. Irregular shedding of the endometrium due to delayed involution of the corpus luteum, when the continuous mixed output of oestrogen and progesterone will result in an endometrium which shows a mixture of late secretory and early proliferative changes at a time when only early proliferative endometrium should be present.
3. Persistence of the corpus luteum is a more exaggerated form of the last-mentioned condition. Here the corpus luteum may fail to regress for weeks or months and produces an excess of both oestrogen and progesterone. Menstruation is delayed and heavy. The persistent corpus luteum may rupture causing lower abdominal pain and sometimes intra-peritoneal haemorrhage which simulates ectopic pregnancy and necessitates laparoscopy and laparotomy.
4. Luteal phase defects cause short menstrual cycles, infertility and early abortions. Luteal phase inadequacy can be diagnosed by daily serum progesterone assays which will show low values. Endometrial biopsy in those cases shows secretory endometrium whose development is consistent with the date of the last menstrual period.

Diagnosis of ovulatory bleeding
Diagnosis of ovulatory bleeding depends on obtaining curettings in the post-ovulatory or secretory phase of the cycle. This is difficult when the menstrual pattern is irregular. A basal body temperature chart should be used to establish the time of ovulation if bleeding is not severe enough to require immediate curettage for treatment.

At diagnostic curettage a careful exploration of the uterine cavity with a polyp forceps should also be done and occasionally a hysterogram or ultrasonogram will show a polyp where other methods have failed.

More detailed investigations of ovulatory function include the measurement of FSH and LH by radioimmunoassay throughout the menstrual cycle, vaginal hormonal cytology and examination of the cervical mucus for cyclical changes.

Treatment of ovulatory bleeding

Once anatomical lesions have been excluded and the diagnosis made with as much precision as possible, the gynaecologist can go on to consider whether medical treatment with hormones is justified or whether the patient needs surgery. Bleeding caused by follicular-phase defects, by irregular shedding of the endometrium and by persistence of the corpus luteum will all usually respond to cyclical oestrogen–progesterone therapy which should be continued for six months. Corpus luteum inadequacy should be treated with small doses of progesterone.

If bleeding is severe, prolonged and complete suppression of menstrual bleeding for a year or more may be indicated and in these circumstances long acting progestational drugs such as medroxyprogesterone acetate can be given in depot form. In the pre-menopausal woman, methyltestosterone, 10 mg daily for 56 days, may be an effective treatment but the response is not always reliable even although androgenic effects are not common with this dosage. Antifibrinolytic drugs such as epsilon-aminocaproic acid have been shown to reduce menstrual blood loss but may cause nausea and vomiting and carry a risk of thromboembolism.

Hysterectomy, as has already been said, may be the correct treatment for the older woman but the decision to perform this operation during reproductive years depends on the severity of the bleeding, the response to hormone treatment and the patient's desire for future children. Hysterectomy should not be performed for dysfunctional bleeding in adolescents or women in their early twenties unless as a desperate, life-saving measure.

THE MENOPAUSE

The definition of the menopause is the cessation of menstruation. In popular use the word 'menopause' has become synonymous with 'climacteric' which means the whole spectrum of physiological and psychological changes surrounding the end of the reproductive phase of life.

Three quarters of women have the menopause between 44 and 50 years, the mean age being 49 years. Increased life expectancy in modern times means that women may expect 20 or 30 years of post-menopausal life.

Endocrine changes

Ovarian function and oestrogen secretion gradually decline. If the decline is more rapid than normal, vasomotor symptoms may be very troublesome. When urinary oestrogen excretion falls below 10 μg/day uterine bleeding ceases. Post-menopausal women continue, however, to show evidence of oestrogenic activity: the origin of this oestrogen is believed to be adrenal. Removal of the ovaries in the post-menopausal woman does not alter the circulating levels of oestrogen which are maintained by a doubling in the rate of the peripheral conversion of adrenal androstenedione to oestrone. With the decrease in production of ovarian oestrogens there is uninhibited production of pituitary gonadotrophins and FSH and LH levels rise.

Other endocrine glands continue to perform normally after the menopause although there is sometimes a decrease in the production of pancreatic insulin which may account for the increased incidence of diabetes in post-menopausal women.

Symptoms
The two classic symptoms of the menopause are vasomotor instability (manifested as hot flushes) and irregularity and eventual cessation of menstruation.

Most other problems at the time of the menopause are caused by stress and anxiety.

Vasomotor symptoms
Oestrogen depletion (or perhaps excess of FSH) disturbs the balance of the hypothalamic-autonomic system and this results in irritability in the blood vessels of the skin, causing the characteristic hot flushes and sweats. The hot flush begins on the chest and spreads quickly over the neck, face and upper limbs. The patient is aware of a blushing sensation which lasts only seconds but may recur many times in the day. Sweating often follows hot flushes. Other vasomotor symptoms include headaches, palpitations and sensations of numbness and tingling.

75 per cent of post-menopausal women experience vasomotor symptoms. Perhaps half of these will experience acute discomfort from these symptoms. Of those patients who have symptoms only about a half seek medical help and if the symptoms are untreated they may persist for one to five years. Vasomotor symptoms can almost always be relieved by treatment with oestrogens.

2. Cessation of menstruation
Although the average age at which menstruation stops is around 50 years, there is wide individual variation. Usually the disappearance of menstruation is gradual. Several episodes of amenorrhea of two

or three months duration are likely to occur before menstruation finally stops. The amount and duration of the periods may remain normal to the end but often they gradually diminish. Neither excessive bleeding nor intermenstrual bleeding are characteristic of the normal menopause and these symptoms should always be viewed as pathological.

Post-menopausal bleeding is defined as vaginal bleeding occurring six months or more after the menopause and should always be assumed to be caused by cancer until proved otherwise.

3. Manifestations of stress and anxiety

There has been a veritable explosion of publicity on the psychology of the menopause and it is widely believed that the 'change of life' has lost its terrors. 'No change' is the current slogan. Despite the prevailing cheerful climate of opinion, women still come to consult their doctors with fears, sometimes explicit, sometimes disguised. A feeling of resentment towards her husband may bring a woman to complain of insomnia, headache, backache or depression, which are all more respectable symptoms than hate. The best way to help such women is not just to send them away with a packet of oestrogens (although these may be of great assistance) but to offer them understanding and support. The doctor may have some difficulty in persuading a woman of 50 that the best is yet to be, for she has much emotional adjustment to make to the loss of youth and the approach of death. She may feel a failure. She may regret lost opportunities in her career and may blame her husband and children for these. She may put undue pressure on her children, trying to make them fulfil her unachieved ambition. She may complain of lack of libido or conversely that she gets no sexual satisfaction because her husband, burdened with business worries, seems to have lost his sex drive. Sexual relationship between husband and wife may need to be completely rebuilt and this can be done very satisfactorily once the problem is recognised.

It has been said that the menopause is a time of loss and that women can only go on to enjoy the next stage of life if they mourn for their lost youth as they would for a loved one, gradually letting his memory go. 'There is no name, with whatever passionate emphasis of love repeated, of which the echo is not faint at last'. When the echo of the past grows faint the new life can begin. At a practical level, the new life can best be encouraged by a new intellectual interest and many women profit from the advice that they should revise their education and seek employment outside of the home.

Metabolic changes

Atherosclerosis
Atherosclerosis is a disease of ageing and there has been considerable argument about whether oestrogens protect post-menopausal women against atherosclerosis and coronary heart disease. Although the administration of exogenous oestrogens to younger women seems to predispose them to circulatory disorders, premenopausal women are more resistant to coronary heart disease than their male contemporaries. The lowered production of natural oestrogens in middle age seems to coincide with an increase in coronary heart disease in women. It seems unlikely that simple oestrogen deficiency is the sole cause of this increased predisposition to coronary atherosclerosis: abnormal secretion of ovarian androgen may also be a factor. The case in favour of the use of oestrogens as a prophylaxis against coronary artery disease is not convincing.

Osteoporosis
Osteoporosis is frequently found in post-menopausal women, increasing in incidence with age. Approximately one per cent of cortical bone mass is lost each year after the menopause. There is now strong evidence that prophylactic oestrogen therapy can prevent and sometimes partially reverse the changes in bone. Treatment to be really effective must be started within a year or two of the menopause and continued into old age. It is not known whether the extent of disability from osteoporosis in the population justifies prophylactic treatment (with any attendant risks it may bring) on a large scale.

Skin changes
A generalised atrophy of skin and mucous membranes gradually takes place after the menopause. The elasticity of connective tissue decreases and the skin wrinkles and dries. Loss of subcutaneous fat results in atrophy of the breasts and vulva. The vaginal skin becomes thin and loses its rugose appearance. Senile vaginitis may cause itch, dyspareunia or blood staining. Also, there may be atrophy of the tissues supporting the urethra which may result in stress incontinence. Local oestrogen therapy often reverses the vaginal changes very effectively but there is little evidence to suggest that oestrogens given by any route preserve skin texture or breast form.

Management of the menopause

What the menopausal woman needs most is education, understanding and reassurance. Despite the intense publicity of recent years, there are still misconceptions to be corrected and it still needs to be emphasised that the end of menstruation is not the end of femininity. There seems no great justification as yet for the wholesale administration of hormones to women who are healthy and are making no complaint for, as has been said, there are doubts surrounding the general use of oestrogens as a prophylaxis against osteoporosis or coronary artery disease. There is every justification, however, for the use of oestrogens to relieve menopausal symptoms. Hot flushes and sweats usually disappear or improve within a few days of starting oestrogen therapy. Other complaints such as headaches may also be relieved, although it would be naive to imagine that simple hormone replacement can cure all the complex symptoms which a menopausal woman may experience.

The gynaecologist would be well advised to concentrate on the cure of specific symptoms which he knows will be relieved by oestrogens.

The woman who has had a hysterectomy and bilateral oophorectomy is a special case – she should receive oestrogens to relieve vasomotor symptoms and treatment can be continued as a logical form of replacement until she has reached post-menopausal age in the confidence that there is no risk of post-menopausal bleeding or uterine cancer. There is now strong circumstantial evidence of an association between oestrogen replacement therapy and endometrial carcinoma, a relationship which some had previously thought doubtful. This finding emphasises the importance of dealing promptly with any bleeding which a woman on hormone replacement therapy may experience. Diagnostic curettage is necessary in all cases.

The aim of oestrogen therapy should be to replace deficiency and to avoid excess.

Patients who are at increased risk of thrombo-embolism such as those with hypertension and diabetes and those with chronic liver disease are best to avoid oestrogens completely. If such women are having severe distress with hot flushes, clonidine 25 to 75 μg daily can produce some relief. Most patients, however, can be prescribed oestrogens, at least in the short term, and there is little doubt of the great clinical benefit produced. Oestrogens are best given orally, so that the dose can be more easily adjusted than with injections or implants. Commonly used preparations are:

1. Conjugate oestrogens   (0·625 to 1·25 mg daily)
2. Oestradiol valerate   (1 to 2 mg daily)
3. Ethinyloestradiol   (0·02 to 0·05 mg daily)

These preparations are usually given in 21 day courses with a 7 day break between each course.

It is difficult to select those patients who should have long term treatment as there is a lack of scientific evidence on this subject.

If the woman has no symptoms at all she should be dissuaded from taking oestrogens, while on the other hand the woman who has deficiency symptoms to a marked degree may require treatment indefinitely.

10

Infertility

Despite world population problems, the desire for reproduction remains a basic human attribute and infertility causes distress to many couples. The causes of infertility vary from country to country and in different social groups. The main variable is the incidence of tubal occlusion caused by infection, either by gonorrhea, tuberculosis or after childbirth or abortion. In general, tubal disease is most common in developing countries and in poor social groups where medical services are not readily available.

Fertility in both men and women is at its maximum in the mid-twenties and, in women, declines rapidly after the age of 30 years. There is some uncertainty about the frequency of intercourse required to achieve pregnancy: twice a week seems the minimum for a reasonable chance of success, and a high rate of pregnancy has been reported after coital frequencies of four or more times weekly. In the absence of contraception, about 60 per cent of women will become pregnant in the first 6 months of marriage, 80 per cent within the first year and 90 per cent within 18 months. It seems reasonable, therefore, to begin the investigation of infertility after a year of normal coitus without contraception.

The clinical management of primary infertility should have a definite plan and a predictable end-point. Most investigations can be completed in 6 months although the couple may need further support after that time.

The traditional 'wait and see' attitude does not satisfy many young people who demand an explanation of their problems within a finite time.

Throughout the investigation both man and woman must be treated as whole, mature people and not as mere appendages to their genital organs. Patients complaining of infertility are often highly sensitive and the doctor should have due regard to the complex psychological and social factors which may be present. Why do the couple want a child? Are they happily married? Is their life together fraught with stress and anxiety about business or financial matters? Is their sex life satisfactory? The answer to these and similar questions may not be apparent at the first interview but such problems may assume increasing importance as the investigation proceeds.

Husband and wife should be interviewed if possible together at the start of the investigation. The paths of male and female investigation diverge thereafter but it is best if there is some firm co-ordination by either the family doctor or the specialist. There is much to be said for joint male/female infertility clinics but hospital arrangements do not always allow these to be set up and men tend to be investigated by urologists while women attend the gynaecologist.

The purposes of an infertility investigation are:

1. To offer an explanation for the infertility.
2. To decide on any necessary and rational treatment.
3. To give a prognosis.

The last of these is the most difficult, because even with modern advances in investigation and treatment there remain between 5 and 10 per cent of healthy married couples in whom no cause for infertility can be discovered by present methods. These people should be told in a realistic manner that the outlook is poor but they should never be deprived of hope. Every experienced gynaecologist knows of pregnancy occurring after adoption and in other circumstances for which there is no rational explanation.

INVESTIGATION OF MALE

Unless the husband is willing to co-operate fully it is futile to investigate the wife unless from the point of view of excluding gynaecological disease and performing any procedure necessary to allow normal intercourse.

History. On taking the history, questions should be asked about childhood illnesses such as mumps or orchitis, occupational hazards including exposure to radio-active substances, hours of work and general life style, consumption of tobacco and alcohol and sexual habits including knowledge of the anatomy of coitus and the delicate questions of impotence and premature ejaculation.

Physical examination. This should be comprehensive. The presence of normal or abnormal male secondary sex characteristics and any evidence of endocrine disorder should be noted. Examination of the genital organs should detect any local factors likely to interfere with testicular temperature such as the wearing of thick or tight underpants and the presence of a varicocele.

Congenital abnormalities such as hypospadias or cryptorchism should also be noted. Failure of descent of the testes leads to azoospermia. Unduly small or absent testes are an indication for chromosomal investigations.

Seminal examination. This is the most important laboratory procedure to be undertaken in the male. The patient should abstain from sex for several days before collection of the specimen. The specimen is obtained by masturbation and is collected in a sterile glass jar to preserve the alkaline pH. The lid of the jar should preferably not be metallic. Rubber or plastic containers should not be used. The laboratory examination should be made within two hours of production of the specimen, so that motility can be studied. An accurate sperm count should also be made and the morphology of the sperms studied on a stained specimen. A normal specimen measures more than 2 ml and contains more than 20 000 000 sperms per ml. More than 75 per cent of the sperms should be motile and there should be less than 25 per cent of abnormal forms. Biochemical tests of the seminal fluid are also of value as they give an index of the function of the seminal vesicles which produce fructose, the prostate which produces acid phosphatase and the epididymis which produces glyceryl phosphoryl choline.

There are many reasons for temporary variations in sperm count and motility and when the findings are unsatisfactory a second specimen should always be examined. Poor motility or numerous abnormal sperm forms are of more serious significance than a low count. If, however, the count is less than 10 000 000 per ml, estimation of FSH, LH and testosterone and tests of thyroid function should be done. Most patients with oligospermia or azoospermia have adequate serum levels of FSH and LH indicating that there is no gonadotrophic deficiency. Serum FSH levels are raised when there is severe destruction of the seminiferous epithelium. Testicular biopsy in men with elevated FSH levels is likely to show germinal cell arrest, sertoli cell syndrome or seminiferous tubule hyalinisation. Fertility cannot be restored in such cases. Testicular biopsy is of little value in men with a sperm count greater than 15 000 000 per ml as minor changes in the epithelium are difficult to assess, histopathology not being an exact science.

Treatment of male infertility

Treatment remains controversial and results are often disappointing. No specific treatment for oligospermia or azoospermia is available at present, but there are a number of measures which may help.

In assessing results in male infertility, it should be remembered that there are great day to day variations in sperm count in normal men and also that the development of spermatozoa takes 70 days, so quick results cannot be expected from any treatment.

General rules of health. General rules of health will be of value to all men, irrespective of the findings on seminal analysis.

1. Excess of alcohol, tobacco and caffeine should be avoided.
2. Fat men should diet to reduce their weight. There should be regular hours of sleep, exercise and work, with adequate leisure and freedom from undue tension.
3. Suitable clothing should be worn and prolonged heating of the testicles (e.g. in chairs or motor cars) should be avoided.
4. Coitus should take place at regular intervals, probably every two or three days. Both excessive coitus and prolonged continence have an adverse effect on the quality of the semen.

Surgical treatment. This is indicated when a varicocele is found in association with subnormal values on seminal analysis. It is claimed that ligation of a varicocele will improve sperm production in 50 to 70 per cent of men treated.

Surgical correction of hypospadias may sometimes be necessary.

Obstruction of the vas deferens is sometimes diagnosed in men with azoospermia, normal serum FSH and LH levels and a normal testicular biopsy and surgical correction may be attempted (epididymovasostomy) but results are poor.

Hormone treatment. This has been extensively employed in various forms without outstanding success. Large doses of testosterone depress spermatogenesis but improved sperm counts and motility have been reported following the use of mesterolone (a mild oral androgen which does not suppress gonadotrophin levels) and fluoxymesterone a slightly more powerful androgen.

Gonadotrophins are indicated as replacement therapy for men with hypopituitarism, e.g. after hypophysectomy, but are otherwise of doubtful value.

Clomiphene has also been used but there is no proof of its efficacy.

Clear and decisive advice. Advice should be given to the husband on conclusion of all necessary investigations. Where there is reasonable hope of fertility, encouragement should be given but if the man appears hopelessly infertile this should be stated clearly. Compassion and understanding on the part of the doctor will help both man and wife to adjust their lives to the facts and to maintain their marriage. Some couples may wish to adopt a child, others may ask for A.I.D., while others may prefer to remain childless.

INVESTIGATION OF FEMALE INFERTILITY

The investigation begins with a general gynaecological history taken in the usual way, including details of previous illnesses and operations, menstrual history, including age at menarche, regularity of menstruation and presence or absence of pain. A general idea should be obtained of the woman's personality and questions should be asked about her mode of life and work. Brief details should then be obtained about the history of her sex life and marriage. These can be amplified in a more meaningful way after the initial clinical examination is performed. It is important to proceed to pelvic examination without unnecessary delay because the patient's reaction to this procedure will give the gynaecologist a great deal of insight into her attitude to sexual matters. It is rather surprising that despite the proliferation of information about sex, a considerable number of marriages are infertile merely because penetration of the vagina has never occurred. In addition to discovering problems related to coitus the gynaecologist may note other abnormalities such as evidence of vaginal infection or the presence of a vaginal septum or double cervix at the initial pelvic examination.

It has already been stressed that the correct approach in the management of infertility is to treat the whole patient, or preferably both patients – husband and wife – but at this stage in the discussion it is convenient to adopt an anatomical approach and consider the different areas in which a cause for infertility may be found together with the relevant investigations can conveniently be conducted in a pattern which roughly follows the anatomical order.

Vulva and vagina
In this region the main problem is dyspareunia and vaginismus. There is seldom any anatomical abnormality to account for this syndrome and the problem is really a psycho-sexual one. It is of the utmost importance that the gynaecologist should approach the examination of the patient with the greatest skill and discretion. If he gains her confidence at this stage, much may be done in the way of treatment. If she feels that she will be hurt or, worse, if she has been hurt, it may be very difficult to establish trust in the doctor's ability to help. A sympathetic but firm attitude and an

economy of words and gesture are advisable. I have found that a simple explanation stating that the problem is due to excessive tension of muscles is easily accepted and forms the basis for treatment. The patient should be told firmly that she can be cured and that this cure will be achieved in part by her own efforts. Treatment with vaginal dilators is then started. This is really an exercise in psychosomatic gynaecology on the doctor's part and it seldom fails. If resort has to be made to surgical procedures, however simple, a great advantage is lost for the patient becomes passive and loses the satisfaction of having cured herself. It is important that, during the period of treatment with dilators (usually a matter of 4 to 6 weeks) no attempt at intercourse is made for if this takes place before the patient has mastered control of her perineal muscles it may be disastrous.

If, after a simple course of treatment with dilators, intercourse is not satisfactory, a deeper psychological cause must be sought.

Cervix

To achieve fertilisation the sperm has to pass through the cervix. Cervical mucus acts as a barrier to sperm except around the time of ovulation when the mucus is thin, translucent and ductile.

The post-coital test was first described by J. Marion Sims in 1866. Mucus is aspirated from the endocervical canal within 12 hours of coitus one or two days before ovulation. The presence of 10 or more progressively motile sperm per high power field (200 ×) is considered satisfactory. The post-coital test is the only infertility test which examines both partners simultaneously. It provides information on the quality of the sperm (a satisfactory test sometimes avoiding the need for semen analysis), the properties of the cervical mucus and the couple's coital technique. A negative post-coital test associated with normal seminal analysis suggests ineffective coital technique due to such causes as incomplete penetration, premature ejaculation or malposition of the cervix.

The post-coital test is widely used in the investigation of infertility but lack of standardisation makes it difficult to interpret the results obtained by various authors. In-vitro sperm-mucus penetration tests (in which samples of semen and cervical mucus are mixed and the penetration of the sperms into the mucus is observed) are complementary to post-coital tests but are not a substitute for them. In-vitro tests are useful when poor post-coital tests are obtained despite proper timing and technique and normal seminal analysis.

When both the post-coital and sperm penetration tests are

abnormal 'cervical mucus hostility' may exist, when the mucus may be deficient, unduly thick, or lethal to sperm. The lethal effect on sperm may be a manifestation of an immune response.

Sperm penetration of cervical mucus may sometimes be improved by giving oestrogens (e.g. 0·01–0·02 mg ethinyloestradiol) for a week before ovulation. Artificial insemination with the husband's semen (AIH), injected into the vagina or cervical canal, may be effective in overcoming cervical hostility. Intrauterine injection of semen can cause painful spasms and should not be done.

Examination of cervical mucus and post-coital tests are easy to perform, require no apparatus other than a microscope and provide results which can be immediately interpreted.

Uterus

Congenital absence of the uterus is a rarity but the possibility should be remembered when the patient is first examined. A rudimentary vagina may be present where there is no uterus. This may occur in a genetic female (where the buccal smear is a chromatin-positive) or in the testicular feminisation syndrome (where the buccal smear is chromatin-negative).

The commonest congenital anomalies of the uterus are various forms of duplication and these are associated more with recurrent abortions than with primary infertility. Some women with double uteri have perfectly normal fertility. Operations aimed at constructing a normal, single uterine cavity may sometimes be indicated in patients with double uteri who are infertile or have recurrent abortions.

Fibroids may also produce gross distortion of the uterine cavity but multiple uterine fibroids are seen in pregnancy often enough to make one doubt whether fibroids really cause infertility. On the other hand, it has been reported that 50 per cent of infertile women with fibroids will become pregnant following myomectomy.

Hysterography with a radio-opaque dye is the best way of defining abnormalities of the uterine cavity. Hysteroscopy may be useful in identification of intrauterine adhesions. The main object of study in the uterus is, of course, the endometrium. In recent years the electron microscope has been used to observe the changes during the menstrual cycle and histochemical methods have increased knowledge of hormones and enzymes, but histology remains the basic technique for evaluating the endometrium. Examination of the premenstrual endometrium gives presumptive evidence of ovulation, evidence about luteal function and may diagnose disease. The biopsy should be taken about two days before menstruation when accurate dating is possible and an index of the entire luteal function is given. A luteal phase defect may be associated with primary infertility as well as with recurrent early abortions. It is diagnosed by inadequate development of the endometrium and may be corrected by treatment of the progesterone. The most important disease diagnosed by endometrial biopsy is tuberculosis. Tuberculous endometritis is always secondary to tuberculous salpingitis and the prognosis for fertility is very poor. In a typical case the characteristic granulomatous histological pattern, with giant cells and tubercles, is seen, but in some instances the appearances are less diagnostic. A sample of endometrium should always be sent for culture and guinea-pig inoculation so that the diagnosis can be made certain.

Various techniques are used for endometrial biopsy. Some gynaecologists perform it as an outpatient procedure on the conscious patient using a fine curette or a suction apparatus. Others prefer to combine it with examination of the pelvic organs under anaesthesia, pointing out that passage of instruments into the nulliparous uterus may sometimes be difficult.

The Fallopian tubes

The Fallopian tubes are more than passive channels through which the ovum is transferred to the uterus. The ampulla and fimbriae pick up the ovum from the site of ovulation; it is transported by the cilia of the endosalpinx to the site of fertilisation; the sperm is transported in the opposite direction, towards the ovum; fertilisation takes place; the zygote is nourished and matured and finally transported to the uterine cavity. Some cases of unexplained sterility may be caused by failure in the hormonal control of this delicate mechanism. Many cases of sterility are certainly caused by blockage of the Fallopian tubes by inflammation. The proximal and interstitial parts of the tube have thick muscular walls and a very narrow lumen and are easily occluded. About a third of infertile patients suffer from some form of tubal damage, the incidence of which obviously increases with a greater incidence of veneral disease and post-abortal sepsis.

While recognising the complexity of the functions of the Fallopian tube, the gynaecologist can do little more in the way of clinical investigation than to detect patency and motility.

Tubal patency and motility can both be demonstrated by *uterotubal insufflation* with carbon dioxide, the test first described by Rubin in 1920 and still used by many gynaecologists as the primary form of tubal investigation. The main error in the performance of the test is leakage of gas from the cervix. A negative result may indicate tubal spasm rather than organic disease and a positive result may sometimes be associated with infertility if there are adhesions around the tube or endometriosis. These faults do not necessarily indicate that this test should be abandoned, for other methods also have their defects. *Hysterosalpingography* has replaced tubal insufflation completely in some centres, while in others it is used as a secondary procedure. Screening under image intensification should show whether the tubes are patent. This test is not always easy to perform and can sometimes be very unpleasant for the conscious patient, especially if performed by someone relatively inexpert in practical gynaecology.

Laparoscopy is now often chosen as the initial investigation of tubal function. Its advocates maintain that 'seeing is believing' and that no other test can match direct inspection and hydrotubation with dyes like methylene blue. There is no doubt, however, the laparoscopy is a potentially dangerous, indeed potentially fatal procedure. Another disadvantage is that there are long waiting lists for laparoscopy in many hospitals. Some gynaecologists reserve it for patients in whom other tests are unsatisfactory or for those who are strongly suspected of having tubal blockage, when it is useful in deciding whether to proceed with tubal surgery. Forms of minor surgery such as division of adhesions and diathermy of endometriosis are sometimes performed through the laparoscope though their value in the treatment of infertility is difficult to assess.

When the delicate lining of the tube has been damaged by inflammation, surgical operations (whether re-implantation, re-anastomosis, salpingolysis or salpingostomy) have a very poor chance of restoring fertility. Such operations should only be performed at the patient's particular request, after explaining the chances of success frankly to her. Despite the relative improbability of becoming pregnant, the patient may feel that she must 'do everything possible' and her mind may not be at rest until the operation is performed.

The ovaries

The ovaries show evidence of inadequate function in 10 to 15 per cent of infertile patients, who either fail to ovulate at all or have an inadequate luteal phase. There are many tests for the detection of ovulation; the first four have the advantage of being simple, relatively cheap and generally reliable clinically.

The biphasic basal body temperature graph (BBT) is simplicity itself, if the patient is reasonably intelligent and co-operative. The temperature is taken orally as soon as the woman wakes each morning and before she moves about, eats, drinks or smokes. The low point occurs at or about the day of ovulation, thereafter the temperature rises in the second half of the cycle to a plateau higher than that in the first half. This rise is associated with the activity of the corpus luteum.

Cervical mucus tests need only a simple microscope. In the first phase of the cycle, oestrogenic activity is associated with a characteristic fern pattern on microscopic examination of the dried mucus. There is increased amount and fluidity of the mucus at the time of ovulation followed by a decrease in amount and absence of fern formation during the second half of the cycle.

Endometrial biopsy has already been discussed. Subnuclear vacuolation is the first sign of ovulation. Well developed secretory changes in the premenstrual phase usually indicate satisfactory progestational activity.

Vaginal cytology shows the response of the vaginal cells to the different ovarian hormones. Smears taken at regular intervals throughout the menstrual cycle give a useful index of ovarian function if a skilled cytologist is available to interpret the results.

Methods which depend upon complicated hormone analysis are expensive and are not universally available, but they have added a great deal to knowledge about ovarian function.

Urinary oestrogen excretion has been used for more than 20 years. The oestrogen peak in the cycle occurs just before ovulation. Daily urinary collections are an inconvenience to the patient and, until automated methods became available they were cumbersome to perform in the laboratory.

Sensitive radio-immunoassay has enabled estimations of serum FSH, LH, total gonadotrophins and prolactin to be standardised and these tests have greatly increased knowledge about ovarian function. Less than 0·5 ml of serum is required for each assay, which means that many hormones can be measured at the same time from a 5 to 10 ml sample of blood. The differences between normal levels of FSH and LH and the high levels associated with ovarian failure are easy to distinguish, but the difference between normal and low levels of FSH and LH are often small and difficult to interpret. The secretion of gonadotrophins is episodic: the most notable variation is the sharp LH peak occurring at ovulation. In clinical practice, therefore, serial samples are necessary so that the rise and fall of the various hormones can be observed. Infertile women whose other investigations have shown no abnormality may, on serial hormone testing, show interesting variations, particularly those which indicate inadequacy of the corpus luteum.

Sonar, using grey-scale imaging techniques provides an interesting, direct and atraumatic method of observing the physical changes in the ovary associated with ovulation. Serial measurements of the ovary throughout the cycle show increasing follicular diameters to about 20 mm before ovulation, followed by a sharp decrease thereafter. This method has great potential value in monitoring the response of the ovary to hormone treatment.

Surgical treatment of ovarian disorders in infertility has little place except in cases of the Stein–Leventhal syndrome, where wedge resection of the ovaries is alleged to result in a restoration of ovulation in 70 to 80 per cent of cases. Wedge resection seems to be associated with a fall in the level of androgen production from the ovary. A disadvantage to wedge resection is that it may (like all operations on the pelvic organs) produce tubo-ovarian adhesions which themselves can cause infertility.

Induction of ovulation by medical means is the most effective way of treating ovarian disorders which cause infertility. The diagnosis of anovulation or defective luteal phase should have been made before starting treatment; it should be certain that the patient has no other medical disorder (e.g. pituitary tumour, thyroid disease) which should be treated first; her Fallopian tubes should have been shown to be patent and her husband not hopelessly infertile. It is obviously nonsense to start treatment aimed at the ovary without first having the basic information about the woman's fertility problem.

Clomiphene citrate is a non-steroid compound consisting of a mixture of cis – and trans – isomers each bound to citric acid. The isomers have different biological properties and this means that commercially available clomiphene has both oestrogenic and anti-oestrogenic properties. Clomiphene can induce ovulation in about 70 per cent of anovulatory women and is an easy drug to prescribe and to take. The usual dosage is 50 mg daily for 5 days beginning on day 5 of the menstrual cycle. If response to this dosage is poor it may be increased by 100 mg daily for 5 days in the next cycle. The maximum safe dose is 200 mg daily. The risks associated with clomiphene treatment are *multiple pregnancy* (15 to 20 per cent, compared with 1 to 2 per cent in nature) and *hyperstimulation* of the ovary. This usually presents as lower abdominal pain or dyspareunia associated with ovarian enlargement. Treatment should be stopped at once if these symptoms and signs appear. Sometimes the ovary may rupture and I have seen a patient with a massive intraperitoneal haemorrhage from this cause. The risks of both multiple pregnancy and ovarian hyperstimulation are, however, less with clomiphene than with gonadotrophins and clomiphene should be the initial treatment for inducing ovulation.

Human chorionic gonadotrophin (HCG) is the treatment of choice when a luteinising hormone is required. It is sometimes used to supplement the action of other gonadotrophins or of clomiphene.

Human pituitary gonadotrophin (HPG) will induce maturation of ovarian follicles but this treatment is limited by the supply of human pituitaries.

Human menopausal gonadotrophin (HMG) is extracted from the urine of menopausal women and is thus more readily available. Its potency is also more predictable than that of HCG. Gonadotrophin treatment may be indicated in secondary amenorrhea where function has been ineffectively stimulated by clomiphene.

Gonadotrophin treatment is dangerous because of the dangers of severe hyperstimulation and the very high incidence of multiple births.

Bromocriptine has already been mentioned in connection with the amenorrhea–galactorrhea syndrome for which it is the treatment of choice. A high serum prolactin level should have been demonstrated before starting treatment.

Induction of ovulation by any method is not without problems and dangers. Patients should be carefully investigated and selected before contemplating treatment and the response should be carefully monitored.

11

Contraception, sterilisation and termination of pregnancy

This is not the place for a discussion on the problem of world population. All educated people admit the urgency for successful family planning at personal and world levels. What follows is an account of methods and of advice that can be given to individuals.

Demographers agree that the responsible modern parent should plan a family of two or not more than three children in an effort to replace but not increase world population. Unfortunately this advice does not reach most of the world's population. It is none the less the duty of the gynaecologist to implement it as best he can for his patients, who, of course, usually resort to contraception not because they think the world is over-populated, but for more personal reasons.

CONTRACEPTION

It is the doctor's duty to advise on contraception to those beginning sexual life and also to discuss it with all his obstetric patients after delivery.

The main methods of contraception are known to all my readers and will merely be summarised here, with brief comments.

It has become the practice to express the efficiency of any contraceptive method by the failure rate per hundred woman years. The number of accidental pregnancies is divided by the number of months exposure and multiplied by 1200 (the number of months in 100 years) i.e.,

Failure rate per 100 woman years

$$= \frac{\text{Total accidental pregnancies}}{\text{Total months exposure}} \times 1200$$

Coitus interruptus

The withdrawal of the penis from the vagina when ejaculation is imminent does not need technical advice and involves no expense but may render the sex act rather unsatisfactory. This method is described in the Old Testament (Genesis 38, 9) and is still in common use. It requires good self control and is unsuitable for those men who tend to have premature ejaculation.

It was once thought to produce all sorts of ill-effects in both sexes including pelvic congestion and prostatitis but there is little objective evidence of this.

The failure rate is quoted as between 6 and 16 per 100 woman years.

The rhythm method

The theory on which this is based is that the ovum cannot be fertilised later than 24 hours after ovulation, that sperm do not survive in the female genital tract longer than four days and that ovulation occurs 14 days before the onset of menstruation. Some of these premises may be incorrect.

If the rhythm method is used it is absolutely necessary to keep an accurate menstrual calendar and it may be advisable to have a record of basal body temperature as well. It is said that the method is very highly successful when the date of ovulation is determined by the temperature chart and intercourse is confined to the immediate post-ovulatory period. This limits exposure to about 10 days per cycle and is therefore a rather tedious method for the newly married.

The failure rate is said to be about 24 per 100 woman years.

The condom

The use of a sheath over the penis during intercourse is the most widely used mechanical contraceptive method. The sheath has the added advantage that it acts as an efficient barrier to infection. It is relatively inexpensive and almost universally available. It has become rather less popular in recent years because it sometimes interferes with the coital sensations of both man and woman. Facts in its favour is that it is pharmacologically inert and non-invasive as opposed to its fashionable competitors the pill and the IUCD.

The failure rate is about 14 per 100 woman years.

Vaginal diaphragm

This mechanical method for the woman is a sophisticated type of contraception which requires intelligence and motivation. The diaphragm must be used with spermicidal cream or jelly and the best method is to insert it at night and remove it, cleanse it and reinsert it the following night. In this way it is always in place, maximum protection is insured and the act of intercourse is not interrupted. Like the sheath, it has no systemic effects. If properly fitted it should be completely comfortable. It places the responsibility for family planning with the woman. The failure rate is quoted as 12 pregnancies per 100 woman years but can be as low as 2.

Spermicidal jellies and foams

These should not be used on their own but in combination with occlusive methods.

The intrauterine contraceptive device (IUCD)

Most IUCDs are made of polythene or nylon in form of spirals, loops, bows, shields or rings. Most of the devices are inert. Some devices incorporate copper which may have a toxic effect but seems to be associated with little in the way of clinical trouble and more recently others have been devised which incorporate a slowly released progestogen.

The IUCD does not demand a high degree of motivation. Once inserted it can be (and often is) forgotten. It is therefore most suitable for the couple with the lowest income and education. For prolonged contraception the well-tried inert IUCDs remain the devices of choice.

The pharmacologically active devices (copper or progestogen) need to be changed at least every 2 years.

Copper devices are small, have a lower expulsion rate and cause fewer effects which demand their removal and hence they have become popular in recent years.

Contra-indications to the use of the IUCD include pelvic inflammatory disease, pregnancy, abnormal uterine bleeding, fibroids and a history of Caesarean section or other operation involving the uterine cavity. Some gynaecologists prefer not to use the IUCD in the nullipara as it may flare up pelvic inflammatory disease and cause subsequent sterility.

The incidence of pelvic inflammatory disease and of deaths from septic abortion are both increased in women wearing the IUCD. The normal vagina contains many bacteria but none are found above the cervical canal and the normal uterine cavity is sterile. Bacteria *are* found, however, in the uterine cavity in women who wear IUCDs with tails. It is probably that the tail acts as a route for infection and that therefore a return to a tailless device as originally recommended by Grafenberg may be desirable.

Menorrhagia is the commonest problem encountered by users

of the IUCD and is the usual reason for requesting its removal. There is a risk of perforating the uterus when inserting the device and sometimes the device disappears at a later date. It can often be recovered from within the uterine cavity by exploration with polyp forceps but if it seems to be outside the uterus an attempt should be made to locate it by X-ray, sonar or laparoscopy. It should be removed by whatever method is appropriate.

Pregnancy occurring with an IUCD *in situ* is reported to be associated with an increase in complications, mainly abortions some of which were in the second trimester. The risk of ectopic pregnancy is said to be increased.

When a woman is found to be pregnant with an IUCD *in situ* (which occurs not uncommonly – perhaps 3 per cent of wearers) the question of termination may arise and also the question of whether the device should be removed or left alone. These are practical questions which the gynaecologist and patient must decide for themselves.

Oral contraceptives

The literature on the contraceptive pill is so vast that it is very difficult to make any sensible comment in a short presentation such as this. It is said that there are 50 million women taking the pill. This is a testimony to its ease, effectiveness and popularity.

Types of oral contraceptive
There are three main types:

1. Combined oestrogen and progestogen, usually taken for 21 days each month, repeating the course after an interval of seven days, whether or not bleeding has occurred.
2. Sequential pills consist of an oestrogen taken for 15 days followed by a progestational agent combined with oestrogen for 5 days. These pills are unreliable in suppressing ovulation and involve taking a high dose of oestrogen.
3. Progestogen only pills give a low dosage of a progestational agent and are taken continuously without a break. They are liable to give rise to irregular bleeding but may be used in some patients for whom oestrogen in any form is contra-indicated.

For all practical purposes the combined oestrogen and progestogen preparations are the only method worth serious consideration. When taken correctly they are virtually 100 per cent effective in controlling conception.

Mode of action

The contraceptive pill acts by suppressing ovulation and produces a pseudo-decidual reaction in the endometrium which discourages implantation. Suppression of ovulation is produced by inhibition of the hypothalamic releasing factors, thus blocking pituitary gonadotrophin activity. The progestational agents inhibit the preovulatory LH surge while the oestrogen inhibits FSH.

Prescribing the pill

All women should have a medical examination before the pill is prescribed and this is usually the province of the general practitioner or the doctor at the family planning clinic. A careful history should include any evidence about contra-indications to taking the pill such as previous thrombosis or embolism, jaundice, breast cancer and oligomenorrhea. Physical examination should include weighing the patient, looking for varicose veins, palpation of the breasts and recording of the blood pressure. Pelvic examination should exclude gross abnormalities of the uterus and adnexa and a cervical smear should be taken. The patient should be instructed clearly on the use of the pill and told that it will only be successful if the instructions are followed. The number of varieties of combined pill available is legion. In general, it is best to prescribe one with a low oestrogen dosage such as 30 micrograms, although low-dose pills should be avoided with patients who are thought to be unreliable in pill-taking. Some form of follow-up is desirable for patients who are on the pill and this should include an annual cervical smear, breast examination and recording of blood pressure. After a confinement the pill can be re-started in the sixth postpartum week or earlier if the patient is not breast feeding. After an abortion the pill can be started in a few days, once all bleeding has stopped.

Complications

The most serious complication reported in association with oral contraception is thrombo-embolic disease. The public are now as well aware of this as they are of the link between smoking and lung cancer and it is sometimes a reason given by women for abandoning the pill. A recent investigation on mortality among users of oral contraceptives in Britain showed that the death rate from diseases of the circulatory system in women who had used oral contraceptives was five times that of controls who had never used them. The risk appeared to increase with age, cigarette smoking and duration of contraceptive use.

The studies, although of great importance, were too small to allow precise conclusions to be reached about the over-all risk of using oral contraceptives. Moreover, while the investigation was in progress there was a progressive reduction in the amount of oestrogen in the contraceptive pills on the market and some preparations containing the progestogen, megestrol acetate, were removed from sale. These changes may have altered the risks.

It would seem, however, reasonable to discourage women over the age of 35 from using the pill especially if they are cigarette smokers. It does not seem justifiable to alarm young women for whom the pill is the ideal contraceptive. Compared to the risks involving the circulatory system, other disadvantages associated with the pill are fairly minor but they may be tedious for the patient and make her want to change her form of contraception.

Some women tend to put on excess weight while on the pill and may have difficulty in controlling it by dieting. Obesity is a hazard to health and predisposes women to circulatory complications. Nausea and migraine are experienced by some and may be related to oestrogen dosage – the pill with the lowest amount of oestrogen should be prescribed for these patients. Depression and lack of libido are thought to be associated with the higher dose pills, but these symptoms may have many and complex causes. Scanty or absent periods may distress some patients and may be a sign of excessive depression of ovarian activity: it is probably unwise to prescribe the pill for patients with oligomenorrhea especially if future fertility is desired. 'Break-through bleeding' is sometimes a nuisance but usually settles within a few months.

Advantages of the pill

The advantages of the pill do not tend to be stressed in either the medical or lay press. It is bad news which hits the headlines. There is no doubt that the pill, properly taken, is the most efficient contraceptive available and is probably ideal for most healthy women under the age of 35. For many women it has abolished the problems of dysmenorrhoea and menorrhagia and has improved their lives enormously.

Long-acting injectable steroids

A single intramuscular injection of medroxyprogesterone acetate 150 mg will inhibit ovulation and menstrual function for three months. The most common indication for this treatment is a temporary measure in association with rubella vaccination. Injections may also be the method of choice for patients who cannot take the pill reliably because of mental retardation.

Sterilisation

When a woman comes with a request for sterilisation the most important duty of the gynaecologist is to ensure that her motives are clear, that she understands the nature of the operation, its risks and its probable irreversibility. The second duty of the gynaecologist is to choose the correct method for his patient e.g. laparoscopic sterilization for some, hysterectomy for others. The third duty of the gynaecologist is to perform the chosen procedure (usually an elective operation on a healthy woman) efficiently and with minimal risk to his patient. Medical and obstetric indications for sterilisation are comparatively few, but more and more women are requesting the operation for the simple reason that they do not wish any more children at any time. It is essential therefore that the patient should be, as the lawyers say in respect of wills 'of a sound and disposing mind', i.e. that she should know what she is asking for and be firm in her decision. She should not take this decision at a time when her reason is clouded by emotion. Patients who are sterilised when young, when in a state of marital unhappiness, at childbirth, in the puerperium or in the post-abortal period are those who most often live to regret the decision.

No sterilisation operation should be performed without the woman's informed consent in writing and it is advisable to have her husband's written consent also. The gynaecologist must be convinced that sterilisation has real advantages over other contraceptive methods for her and should explain his intention and reasons for sterilisation to the woman's general practitioner. As has already been said the patient must accept that the operation usually has a permanent effect. At the same time she must know that it is not possible to guarantee that there will be no conception after sterilising operations, short of total hysterectomy and bilateral salpingo-oophorectomy.

An interview with a woman who requests sterilisation is a delicate matter. The facts must be put clearly but her confidence should not be destroyed by emphasising unduly the risks and possible failure of the operation.

In choosing the type of operation the surgeon should aim to produce the necessary effect without destruction of tissue.

The damage inflicted by laparoscopic tubal diathermy, for example, is always greater than it appears to be at the time of operation and the tube may in some cases be almost completely destroyed. This makes this technique less than ideal for the young woman who, however adamant may seem her resolve for sterilisation, may seek reversal at a later date. For the young patient a more conservative method such as the use of rings or clips may be better.

For the older patient who has troublesome gynaecological symptoms or a diseased uterus a tubal sterilising operation may be completely inappropriate and hysterectomy either abdominal or vaginal may be the correct treatment. It has been said that nearly one in five of women who have tubal sterilising operations need to have a hysterectomy for one reason or another at a later date. Hysterectomy carries an undoubted mortality and morbidity, but it removes further menstrual problems and the possibility of uterine cancer. Women often welcome the prospect of hysterectomy rather than many years of hormonal contraception. Before making the decision to choose hysterectomy there must be a full explanation to the patient, time to reflect on the decision and eventually absolutely clear motivation. It is seldom wise for the gynaecologist to apply any pressure on a woman to have a hysterectomy. The various forms of sterilisation in common use may be summarised as:

Sterilisation as a primary procedure
1. *Laparotomy*. Numerous techniques in use. Object should be to divide the tube and separate the divided ends.
2. *'Mini-Laparotomy'*. Access to the tubes is gained through a proctoscope or similar instrument inserted via a small suprapubic incision.
3. *Posterior colpotomy*, exposing the tubes via the pouch of Douglas.
4. *Laparoscopy*. At present most popular method. Tubes are occluded by bands or clips in young patients for whom reversal may later be requested. In older women with no menstrual disturbance bilateral tubal diathermy is the usual method. It carries the danger of diathermy injury to bowel and other viscera but none the less is the most popular technique.
   All laparoscopic techniques require skill and experience which can only be gained by practical instruction at the hands of an expert.

Sterilisation in association with another operation
1. *Caesarean section*. This may be a well considered decision taken in advance, particularly in the case of a woman who has had two or three previous Caesarean sections, but the decision about sterilisation in association with section should not be arrived at

in a hurry: in an emergency, sterilisation is often better post-poned.
2. *Termination of pregnancy.* Salpingocleisis can be performed when hysterotomy is done to terminate pregnancy. Hysterotomy is a much less common operation now. It is doubtful whether the time of termination is the right time to perform an ir-reversible operation on the tubes.
3. *Pelvic floor repair.* If the patient complains of prolapse and also requests sterilisation, vaginal hysterectomy may be ideal.
4. *Abdominal hysterectomy* has already been mentioned as a possible primary method of sterilisation but the issue may arise in another form as, for example, in discussing with a patient whether she should have myomectomy or hysterectomy as treatment for fibroids.

Male sterilisation
Male sterilisation by vasectomy is becoming increasingly popular but this is not the place to discuss it. Wives of men who have had vasectomies should know that other contraceptive methods need to be employed until two negative semen tests have been obtained at 8 and 12 weeks after the operation.

Much has been written about the late effects of female sterilisa-tion and the incidence of such problems as dysfunctional uterine bleeding, emotional regret, dyspareunia, decreased libido and dysmenorrhea. There is, however, a lack of objective information on these topics as hitherto there has been no prospective study, no controls, no complete follow-up study and such results as have been reported have been very variable.

According to some workers 40 per cent of women experience increased menstrual loss after laparoscopic tubal diathermy as com-pared with 20 per cent after sterilisation by laparotomy. Such results are difficult to interpret.

What is clear, however, is that the gynaecologist's plain duty is to make sure that his patient is well informed about sterilisation and its effects and that her resolve is firm. In this way there is less likelihood of making mistakes which will bring future unhappiness.

Termination of pregnancy
The law on termination of pregnancy in Scotland, England and Wales is set out in the Abortion Act of 1967 which states that:
A person should not be guilty of an offence under the law relating to abortion when a pregnancy is terminated by a registered medical

practitioner, if two registered medical practitioners are of the opinion, formed in good faith that:

1. The continuance of the pregnancy would have involved risk to the life of the pregnant woman greater than if the pregnancy were terminated.
2. The continuance of the pregnancy would have involved risk of injury to the physical or mental health of the pregnant woman greater than if the pregnancy were terminated.
3. The continuance of the pregnancy would have involved risk of injury to the physical or mental health of the existing child(ren) of the family of the pregnant woman greater than if the pregnancy were terminated.
4. There was a substantial risk that if the child had been born it would have suffered from such physical or mental abnormalities as to be seriously handicapped.

IN CASE OF EMERGENCY

5. It was necessary to save the life of the pregnant woman; *or*
6. It was necessary to prevent grave permanent injury to the physical or mental health of the pregnant woman.

It is important that gynaecologists should know what the law says but it is immediately obvious that wide variations in interpretation are possible. Disputes on the Abortion Act tend to generate more heat than light and this is not the place for ethical discussion except to make the simple points that abortion involves the destruction of human life and that every woman who contemplates taking such a step deserves a compassionate hearing, efficient and accurate clinical examination, a decision made not in haste but after due reflection and treatment carried out with skill to ensure her present safety and future health.

In Scotland the vast majority of abortions are performed in N.H.S. hospitals and in the years 1972–75 the grounds for abortion notified were:

Grounds for abortion	Number of cases 1972–1975
Risk to life of woman	255
Risk to physical or mental health of woman	27 953
Risk to physical or mental health of existing children	1 374
Risk of abnormality to fetus	432
Emergency cases	11

This clearly shows that the commonest indication for termination was under Clause 2 of the Act which is open to wide interpretation. In recent years much research and clinical effort has gone in to devising simple and safe methods of abortion. These methods have not been entirely successful and abortion remains the greatest single cause of maternal death.

The methods of termination used in Scottish hospitals in the period 1972–75 give a reasonable indication of the main techniques used:

Method of termination	Number of cases 1972–1975
Abdominal hysterotomy	2 529
Vaginal hysterotomy	54
Dilatation and evacuation	4 255
Vacuum aspiration	19 028
Other (including prostaglandins)	4 359

During the period reviewed the number of hysterotomies dropped consistently, while the number of prostaglandin terminations increased.

It is now appropriate to review these techniques in more detail. The earlier a pregnancy is terminated the less risk to the patient. The uterus can be evacuated with much greater ease and safety when it is 8 to 10 weeks size than between 10 and 14 weeks.

The difficulties and dangers involved in later termination are not because of fetal size but because of haemorrhage, infection, cervical laceration and uterine perforation.

The extremity in early termination of pregnancy is exemplified by the so-called 'menstrual aspiration' where vacuum curettage of the uterus is performed within 10 to 18 days of the first missed period. To some this 'ten-minute abortion' seems a convenient social service; to others it seems the ultimate in the trivialisation of human life.

Unfortunately all terminations cannot be done so early and so easily. This applies particularly to cases of fetal abnormality which cannot be diagnosed before 16, 18 or even 20 weeks. Similarly termination may be indicated late in the second trimester of pregnancy because of serious complications such as eclampsia or haemorrhage which threaten the life of the mother.

It is fortunate that developments in pharmacology have led to safer and more efficient methods of mid-trimester abortion using prostaglandins, making hysterotomy a comparative rarity.

Abdominal hysterotomy

In the early years after the passing of the Abortion Act about 20 per cent of legal abortions were carried out by abdominal hysterotomy. In Scotland in 1972 approximately 15 per cent of abortions were done by this method but by 1975 the figure had fallen to 3 per cent. Cases still arise where abdominal hysterotomy, because of its immediate effect or because of the need to perform some other abdominal operation at the same time, remains the method of choice. At operation, the bladder is displaced down off the anterior uterine wall and a vertical midline incision is made as low in the uterus as possible. The gestation sac is evacuated digitally and the uterus is repaired.

Abdominal hysterotomy is associated with a substantial postoperative morbidity and late complications may include uterine rupture in a subsequent pregnancy or labour, particularly if the incision in the uterus has been badly sited and inadequately repaired.

Implant endometriosis is another complication of abdominal hysterotomy and further surgery may be required to remove an endometrioma.

Vaginal hysterotomy

Although still occasionally performed, vaginal hysterotomy is now little more than a curiosity. In the pre-antibiotic era it was used for evacuating a potentially infected gestation sac when the uterus was more than 12 weeks size, in order to avoid opening the peritoneal cavity.

Instrumental dilation and evacuation

This was the standard method of terminating an early pregnancy before vacuum aspiration was introduced. It can still be used with ease and safety when the uterus is less than 10 weeks size. It should be remembered that dilatation of the cervix (whether preliminary to vacuum aspiration or instrumental curettage) is a dangerous procedure which may result in the immediate risk of haemorrhage and the late risk of cervical incompetence and recurrent unsuccessful pregnancy. If possible the cervix should be stretched until a finger can be introduced into the uterus. The index finger of the right hand explores the uterine cavity while the left hand, on the abdomen, grasps the uterine fundus. 'The finger is the safest curette' and the more tissue that can be removed digitally the better. Gentle instrumental curettage completes the operation.

Vacuum aspiration

Vacuum aspiration is now the most popular method. Again, great care and gentleness, combined with a knowledge of the apparatus is essential. Immediately after aspiration the uterus should be explored gently with ovum forceps and curette to remove any retained fragments.

Vacuum aspiration is very safe, especially if the minimum dilatation of the cervix is employed.

Prostaglandins

Unlike oxytocin, prostaglandins can stimulate uterine activity at any stage of gestation. F prostaglandins (PGF_2 α) were the first form used for the induction of abortion but have been abandoned because of the vomiting and diarrhoea they caused.

PGE_2 causes rather less in the way of gastrointestinal effects but, in the large doses needed to induce abortion neither oral nor intravenous administration is entirely suitable. Fortunately, prostaglandins are locally acting hormones and can be conveniently instilled into the uterus by the extra-amniotic route. The method is simple and atraumatic: the cervix is exposed and a Foley catheter is introduced so that the balloon lies just inside the internal os.

PGE_2 can be given in a test dose of 50 μg followed by 200 μg two hourly, or else an equivalent dose can be given by a continuous variable-rate infusion pump. This method is usually successful in producing abortion within 24 hours. Once contractions are established, oxytocin may be added to enhance the effect of prostaglandins and, after spontaneous passage of products of conception, instrumental evacuation of the remainder is usually easy.

Intra-amniotic injection of prostaglandins may be given through the abdominal wall. The intra-amniotic injection of PGE_2 2·5 mg plus 80 g urea is a powerful abortifacient but as with other hypertonic solutions, there is a risk of causing disseminated intravascular coagulation.

Recently, trials have been made of local administration of prostaglandins in a viscous gel which acts as a slow-release vehicle, delaying the absorption of PGE_2. A single extra-amniotic injection of 1·5 mg PGE_2 in viscous gel seems to provide optimum efficiency combined with avoidance of excessive vomiting.

Other methods of termination

Other methods of termination have been rendered obsolete by the techniques described above. The use of local abortifacients such as laminaria tents and utus paste stands condemned because of the risk to life.

Intra-amniotic injections of hypertonic solutions – saline, glucose or urea – have also fallen into disrepute because of sepsis and other complications.

Complications

Complications of induced abortion are possible, no matter what method is used. They can be classified under the general headings of trauma, infection and haemorrhage.

Trauma. Trauma may be in the form of vaginal or cervical laceration or uterine rupture. Bladder, ureters and bowel may also sustain damage.

Infection. Infection is an ever present risk, increasing with the lack of asepsis and antisepsis which is usually associated with illegal abortion. Endotoxic bacteraemic shock is a life-endangering complication which is particularly prone to arise in cases of abortion. Tubal occlusion and consequent infertility is a common late result of poor abortal sepsis.

Haemorrhage. Haemorrhage may be the result of both trauma and infection or else the result of uterine atomy associated with retained products of conception.

If the mother is Rhesus negative and the fetus Rhesus positive, fetal cells may escape into the maternal circulation. This can be detected by the Kleihauer test or by serum alpha-feto-protein measurement. In these circumstances the mother should be given anti-D gammaglobulin.

12

Infections of the genital tract

The genital tract is a pathway by which it is possible for infection to ascend all the way from the vulva to the ovaries and peritoneal cavity, but normally the acidity of the vagina (pH 4 or 5) prevents this process. The surface cells of the vagina are rich in glycogen from which the Döderlein's bacilli manufacture lactic acid. In addition to Döderlein's bacilli, the normal vaginal flora contains streptococci, staphylococci and diphtheroids. The physiological vaginal discharge is heavier when women are pregnant or are taking the contraceptive pill. Habits of cleanliness help to prevent vulvitis and vaginitis, as would be expected, but the widespread use of nylon underwear in the western countries produces conditions of warmth and moisture which favour the persistence of vaginal infections.

INFECTIONS OF THE VULVA

General skin diseases
Any skin disease may affect the vulva and infection of the hair follicles on the labia majora is not uncommon. Herpes simplex may appear as a painful vesicular lesion. Herpes type II virus may be linked with the development of cervical cancer.

Moniliasis
By far the commonest form of vulvitis is moniliasis which may assume a very chronic form and be associated with extensive skin changes of the 'chronic vulvar dystrophy' type. Biopsy of the vulva may be necessary to exclude pre-malignant change. Moniliasis is often associated with pregnancy or diabetes.

Venereal disease
Venereal disease may present as vulvar lesions. *Syphilis* in the primary stage appears as a small chancre which regresses in a month or so; in the second stage condylomata lata may appear; gummatous

ulcers, characteristic of the third stage, are now rarely seen. *Chancroid*, caused by the Haemophilus Ducrey appears as a painful pustular ulcer.

Lymphopathia venereum is associated with vulvar oedema and ulceration and *granuloma inguinale* with extensive ulceration of the vulva. Both these diseases are characteristic of the tropics; lymphopathia venereum is diagnosed by the Frei test (an antigen–antibody reaction) and granuloma inguinale by the presence of Donovan inclusion bodies on smears. All of these venereal diseases respond to antibiotics.

Bartholinitis

The statement is often made that gonorrhea is the commonest cause of Bartholinitis, but this assertion is seldom demonstrated in clinical practice in Britain. Infection with coliform organisms is probably more common. Acute infection may be associated with abscess formation and chronic infection with occlusion of the duct and consequent formation of a cyst. Bartholin's cysts are best treated by marsupialisation, which minimises the risk of recurrence.

INFECTIONS OF THE VAGINA

The treatment of vaginitis forms a large part of routine gynaecological practice and the main types of vaginal infections and their treatment are so well known that they will only be mentioned briefly.

Trichomoniasis

Trichomoniasis is probably spread by sexual intercourse and reinfection is particularly liable to occur just after menstruation when the pH of the vagina is increased. The diagnosis is made by recognition of the typical frothy yellow-green vaginal discharge with 'strawberry spots' – small granular petechiae – on the posterior fornix and cervix and by seeing the trichomonads themselves (flagellated oval organisms with a characteristic shivering movement) on high power microscopy of a drop of discharge suspended in saline at body temperature. The most commonly used treatment is Metronidazole 200 mg thrice daily for the patient and her male partner.

Moniliasis

Moniliasis is probably more common than trichomonal infection and causes more vulvar irritation and excoriation. There is a thick cheesy discharge and thrush-like patches are seen on the vaginal wall. On microscopy fungal strands or mycelia can be identified. The monilia (or candida) albicans thrives in the presence of carbohydrate and this explains the increased incidence in pregnancy and in diabetics. Antibiotics destroy the organisms which normally check the growth of the monilia fungus, so moniliasis can easily become established after the patient has had a course of antibiotic treatment. Once infection with monilia occurs it is difficult to eradicate, for the organisms lodge in the folds of the vaginal epithelium and in the cervix. The well-established and still generally effective treatment of moniliasis vaginae is the local application of Nystatin. Two Nystatin vaginal tablets are inserted nightly for two weeks, continuing the treatment during menstruation. Nystatin cream is used in association with the tablets. If local treatment is not successful it may be because the cervix is acting as a reservoir to infection and should be treated by diathermy conisation or cryocautery.

Gonorrhea

Gonorrhea, despite its increasing prevalence, remains a difficult disease to diagnose in women. A first attack may manifest itself as an acute vaginitis and the typical gram-negative intracellular diplococcus may be easily detected on high-power microscopy of a fresh smear. However, the presence of the gonococcus may be masked by trichomonads or other organisms and if there is no history of contact, no specific search may be made for it in a fresh specimen. The difficulty in diagnosis can be partly avoided by taking 'triple swabs' – urethral, vaginal and cervical – and sending them to the laboratory in a transport medium (e.g. Stuart's medium).

Gonorrhea may spread rapidly in young children who have no resistance because they have not developed the acid vaginal pH. Epidemics of the disease have been recorded from institutions where girls are living in close proximity. The subject of gonorrhea will be discussed further under 'pelvic inflammatory disease'.

Atrophic vaginitis

This may be a source of troublesome symptoms in post-menopausal women. Post-menopausal oestrogen deficiency is accompanied by a reduction in the activity and numbers of Döderlein's bacilli and subsequent invasion of the vagina by normally harmless organisms such as the anaerobic streptococcus. In some women there may be quite profuse discharge; in some there may be bleeding, which of course requires full investigation; in others, dyspareunia is the presenting symptom. Treatment with oestrogens, often given locally in the form of creams, is usually effective.

Foreign bodies

Foreign bodies in the vagina may cause offensive foul-smelling discharge. The most notorious of these is the neglected tampon whose removal can be an unpleasant olfactory experience. Children may sometimes put toilet paper and other material into the vagina with similar results.

PELVIC INFLAMMATORY DISEASE

This is a composite syndrome which is secondary to ascending infection from the vagina and cervix. No symptoms may develop when the infection reaches the uterus but the main symptoms occur when there is extension into the tubes (salpingitis) the ovary (oophoritis) or peritoneum (pelvic peritonitis).

This disease usually begins with an acute episode which may resolve completely with treatment or may go on to a chronic illness with recurrent exacerbations of the inflammatory process.

There are three basic aetiological groups of pelvic inflammatory disease.

1. *Pyogenic.* Infections with streptococci, staphylocci coliforms and the like. This is the type of infection, usually endogenous, which occurs after childbirth or abortion.

2. *Gonococcal.* Gonorrhea is a world wide problem but in Britain pyogenic infections are probably commoner.

3. *Tuberculous.* This may be asymptomatic. Decrease in pulmonary tuberculosis in Western countries has made genital tuberculosis in women a comparatively rare disease.

1. *Pyogenic post-abortal or puerperal infection*

The infection spreads up through the lymphatics and causes a parametritis. There is an interstitial salpingitis with thickening of the tubal wall and a cellular infiltration of the meso-salpinx. The tubal mucosa may remain normal and the possibility of subsequent pregnancy may be unimpaired provided prompt effective treatment is given. Sometimes there may be peritonitis with formation of an abscess in the pouch of Douglas.

The patient with pelvic infection after an abortion (which is the commonest type of pyogenic infection likely to be encountered in modern practice) is fevered, restless and looks ill. She may have rigors. She will have marked lower abdominal tenderness on both sides. On pelvic examination there will be tenderness on moving the cervix and bilateral parametrial thickening. Speculum examination may show a foul vaginal discharge and remnants of products of conception. It is important to bear in mind the possibility of ectopic pregnancy in the differential diagnosis. When there is serious doubt, laparoscopy should be done.

The vascular uterus allows rapid invasion with coliforms and other Gram-negative organisms so that endotoxic bacteraemic shock may sometimes occur. This is discussed below.

Prompt effective antibiotic treatment is the best preventive of endotoxic shock and will minimise the late results of pelvic infection. As soon as an effective blood level of antibiotic has been reached the uterus should be evacuated, for retained products may act as a persistent source of infection. Antibiotics of the tetracycline or cephalosporin groups are widely effective against most of the infecting organisms, while metronidazole seems to be specifically suitable against bacteroides necrophorus.

Specimens should be taken immediately for bacteriological examination but it is important that treatment with a broadspectrum antibiotic should also start immediately without waiting for the bacteriological report. Alterations in treatment can be made once details of sensitivity are known. Response to antibiotics is usually rapid. A good initial choice for the usual post-abortal case would be cephazolin 1 g twice daily.

2. Gonococcal pelvic infection.

The ascending spread of gonorrhea is different from that of the pyogenic organisms usually involved in post abortal infection and this results in important differences in pathology.

The initial focus of infection is usually the cervix but it may sometimes be the urethra or Bartholin's gland. The disease spreads directly along mucosal surfaces and the mucosa of the tube shows the main pathological changes. There is extensive endo-salpingitis with marked hyperaemia, oedema and purulent discharge. Pus escaping from the ends of the tubes may lead to pelvic peritonitis and a pelvic abscess may form. If there is closure of the fimbriated end of the tube the pus is blocked inside and a pyosalpinx forms; as the infecting organisms disappear the pus resolves into a clear fluid and the condition of hydrosalpinx is established.

Involvement of the ovary in the inflammatory process may lead to the formation of a tubo-ovarian abscess. The gonococcus may disappear from the tube within 10 days so that subsequent culture may be sterile even although the tube is extensively diseased. The damage to the tubes may be irreversible and infertility will then result.

Gonococcal pelvic inflammatory disease causes lower abdominal pain and tenderness, fever, nausea, vomiting and tachycardia – the clinical picture already described under 1. Pyogenic post-abortal or puerperal infection. Appendicitis, urinary infection and ectopic pregnancy are the three main conditions to be considered in differential diagnosis. When a woman is admitted to hospital with acute pelvic inflammatory disease which does not seem to be related to childbirth or abortion it is as well to assume that it is due to gonorrhea until proved otherwise. The usual triple swabs from urethra, vagina and cervix should be taken and treatment started with the best available antibiotic for gonorrhea. At present, this is probably oral doxycycline: a starting dose of 300 mg is followed by 200 mg 12-hourly until the pain disappears and then by 100 mg 12-hourly for 14 days.

3. Genital tuberculosis

Genital tuberculosis is always secondary to tuberculosis elsewhere, usually in the lung: the disease spreads through the bloodstream. In the pelvis it is mainly the tubes that are involved. There is a granulomatous salpingitis, with giant and epithelioid cells and there are various degrees of caseation and fibrosis, depending on the acuteness or chronicity of the process.

Endometrial tuberculosis is always secondary to tubal disease; involvement of the endometrium occurs in about half the patients with tuberculous salpingitis. Genital tuberculosis may produce no symptoms whatever in the initial stages. Most patients with this disease come complaining of infertility. In others the picture may be one of pelvic inflammation which has failed to respond to the usual antibiotic treatment.

Curettage is essential for diagnosis and this should be done in the pre-menstrual phase. Specimens of endometrium are sent for histology and for guinea pig inoculation. Tuberculosis does not interfere with ovulation and the intractable infertility with which it associated is, of course, the result of tubal occlusion.

Treatment is by combinations of various anti-tuberculous drugs. One method is to administer streptomycin 1 g daily, isonicotinic acid (INH) 100 mg thrice daily and para-aminosalicylic acid (PAS) 3 g four times daily for three months. The streptomycin is then stopped but treatment with INH and PAS is continued for 18 months.

Curettage, as a test of cure, is done at six monthly intervals.

More recent drugs used in the treatment of tuberculosis include rifampicin and ethambutol: the latter is liable to give rise to eye complications.

Intrauterine pregnancy is rare even after full treatment for tuberculosis because primary tubal damage has usually occurred before the diagnosis is made.

Ectopic pregnancy is more likely to occur and its possibility should always be borne in mind.

Chronic pelvic inflammatory disease from whatever infecting organism may be a disabling condition for the patient and a tedious problem for the gynaecologist.

Some patients with tuberculosis may only be diagnosed when the disease has already become chronic and although tuberculosis is much rarer than formerly its possibility should be remembered in the case of resistant chronic pelvic inflammation. Pre-menstrual curettage will make the diagnosis.

Acute pelvic inflammation, whatever the cause, if not eradicated by primary treatment may subside into subacute or chronic stages. There is a tendency to repeated exacerbations either caused by rein-fection by a sexual partner or by the release of organisms from the cervix. An intrauterine contraceptive device may also provide a persistent channel for ascending infection and it has been shown that the incidence of pelvic inflammation is increased three times or more in women who wear the IUCD as opposed to controls who do not. Unfortunately, the woman with the irresponsible life style for whom the IUCD is the best available contraceptive is also the woman most at risk from pelvic inflammatory disease.

The symptoms of chronic pelvic inflammation are recurrent lower abdominal pain, backache, rectal discomfort, dyspareunia, discharge, dysmenorrhoea and menorrhagia. The clinical signs include tenderness on pelvic examination and various degrees of adnexal thickening or swellings. If a pelvic abscess is present it should be drained by posterior colpotomy and emergency laparotomy may sometimes be necessary for a ruptured tubo-ovarian abscess.

Patients with tubal blockage sometimes ask for an operation to restore their fertility and it can be difficult to dissuade them from persisting with this request although when the tubes are damaged by inflammation there is little prospect of restoring normal function.

The woman whose first pregnancy was terminated for social reasons, who subsequently had her tubes blocked as a result of inflammation, perhaps from wearing an IUCD, and who now passionately desires a child is encountered from time to time in modern gynaecological practice and presents a sad figure. She can be given only a rather dismal prognosis.

Eventually, radical surgery in the form of total hysterectomy and bilateral salpingo-oophorectomy may be required as the ultimate solution to the problem of chronic pelvic inflammatory disease. No surgical procedure less than removal of the uterus, tubes and ovaries is likely to be curative and in this era of hormone replacement therapy castration in a comparatively young woman is not such a disaster as it was in former years. The indications for radical surgery include:

a. Repeated exacerbations of inflammation, not satisfactorily controlled by antibiotics.
b. Persistent pain and dyspareunia.
c. Incapacitating menstrual disorders – dysmenorrhea or menorrhagia.
d. Increase in size of pelvic masses.

Operating on patients with extensive pelvic inflammatory disease can be a formidable procedure, calling for great technical skill.

SEPTIC SHOCK (BACTERAEMIC OR ENDOTOXIC SHOCK)

Shock is defined as inability of the circulatory system to meet the needs of the tissues for oxygen and nutrients and to remove toxic metabolites. Shock may be hypovolaemic, cardiogenic or septic in origin. Patients with pelvic infections, particularly those associated with abortion which are mainly caused by Gram-negative organisms, are at high risk of developing septic shock.

The basic microvascular disturbances are the same in all types of shock. There is decreased tissue perfusion due to arteriolar constriction with increased resistance and venular constriction with decreased capacitance.

In the next stage there is loss of arteriolar constriction but persistence of venular constriction. This gives rise to stagnation, microthrombosis, oedema and cell death in the tissues perfused by these vessels. At this stage, a generalised coagulation disorder may begin. In septic shock, the deterioration in the micro-circulation may occur in minutes due to bacterial endotoxin, a complex lipopolysaccharide which may act as an antigen.

Another probable action of endotoxin is to open all arteriovenous anastomoses and thus to allow the circulation to bypass the affected tissues: this results in a great reduction of perfusion of the micro-vascular bed and consequent cell death.

Knowledge about the nature and action of endotoxin is advancing rapidly and it is now possible to test for endotoxin by mixing it with an amoebocyte extract derived from limulus polyphemus (the horse-shoe crab).

Organisms involved in septic shock
Two-thirds of these are Gram-negative. The most important are:

Coliforms
Klebsiella
Proteus
Ps. pyocyanea
Bacteroides

Gram-positive organisms, involved in the remaining one third of patients include:

Staphylococcus
Streptococcus
Clostridium Welchi

Clinical features of septic shock
Clinical features of septic shock are manifested in three stages. The difficulty in the early diagnosis of this dangerous condition lies in the fact that the patient, to the superficial observer, may look alert and well.

Stage 1. 'Warm Normotension'. The patient may be slightly flushed, may be rather apprehensive but her skin seems well perfused and the arterial blood pressure is normal.

Stage 2. 'Warm Hypotension'. The patient although still very alert seems extremely anxious. She is fevered, flushed and has rapid respirations and pulse. Arterial blood pressure is dramatically low when considered in relation to the patient's appearance.

Stage 3. 'Cold Hypotension'. The patient is now in a state of shock in the traditional sense with peripheral and central circulatory failure. Respiratory dysfunction and failure of gas exchange may lead to the condition of 'shock lung' (see below). Renal failure and hepatic dysfunction may also be present.

Treatment of septic shock
Because of its complex nature and because of the continuous monitoring required septic shock is best treated in a specialised

intensive care unit. Attention to detail is of the greatest importance and sophisticated biochemical and biophysical techniques have proved of great value. When septic shock is diagnosed the patient should be transferred to the intensive care unit wherever possible so that treatment can be started early. The factors which lead towards irreversible shock and death are (i) prolonged duration of shock (ii) failure to eliminate sepsis by operation and (iii) inappropriate antibiotic therapy.

The aims of treatment of septic shock are to stabilise vital functions and to identify and correct specific haemodynamic and metabolic derangements.

Simple preliminary measures may be started right away in the gynaecological ward.

1. Give oxygen by high-concentration mask.
2. Maintain circulatory volume by intravenous plasma.
3. Put in an indwelling catheter to measure hourly urine output.
4. Send blood samples for urea, electrolytes, group and cross-matching, bacteriological culture and coagulation screen.
5. Give intravenous antibiotics. Gentamycin and metranidazole seems the most effective combination at present.
6. A central venous pressure line (CVP) may be set up if there is time but ineffective attempts to do this are time wasting and possibly dangerous. It has been said that CVP monitoring is essential for proper management, but its limitations must be recognised. It reflects the ability of the right side of the heart to cope with the venous return at the moment of measurement. It does not measure blood volume and is an unreliable guide to the infusion of crystalloids. False high values are common.

Once specialist help is available efforts are directed towards maintaining respiration and circulation as soon as possible. Ventilation of the lungs is carried out by tracheal intubation and intermittent positive pressure ventilation. This may help to protect the patient against the insidious development of 'shock lung' where there are consolidation, platelet and leucocyte emboli, fibrin deposition and intra-alveolar haemorrhage and oedema.

The circulation is sustained by intravenous infusion of colloids and crystalloids, by the use of vasodilators such as chlorpromazine and thymoxamine, of positive inotropics like digoxin, dopamine and isoprenaline and of diuretics like frusemide and mannitol. (Frusemide should not be used with cephalosporins – the combination is nephrotoxic.) Monitoring obviously is an important part of the work of the intensive care unit. Continuous electrocardiography, CVP measurement, systemic arterial pressure and core-peripheral temperature gradients all yield valuable information about the cardiovascular system. Respiratory function is monitored by vital capacity, expiratory volume and blood measurements of pH, P_aO_2, P_aCO_2 and base excess or deficit.

Hourly urine output gives an index of renal function. If there are signs of acute tubular necrosis dialysis may be necessary. Antibiotics are the keystone of treatment and as has been said gentamycin and metronidazole seem the best combination at present. In addition to medical treatment of infection, surgery may be needed to eradicate the septic focus. In the gynaecological patient this may involve anything from a simple curettage to a rather hazardous hysterectomy.

The blood coagulation tests are often abnormal but heparinisation is rarely required.

Corticosteroids have long been given in the treatment of endotoxic shock but their value has never been demonstrated on controlled trial. The modern view is that steroids given early may protect against lysosomal enzymes, but are no use unless given in this prophylactic way.

Success in the treatment of endotoxic shock seems to depend on:

1. Early recognition
2. Rapid treatment with effective antibiotics
3. Haemodynamic support
4. Ventilation of lungs
5. Surgical removal of septic focus where necessary.

Observation of these principles has reduced mortality by one half in 10 years in at least one intensive care unit.

13

Endometriosis and fibroids

ENDOMETRIOSIS

Endometriosis is defined as the presence of tissue resembling the endometrium in sites outside the uterine cavity. Adenomyosis, when this tissue is found in uterine muscle, is sometimes described as *endometriosis interna* while *endometriosis externa* is the term used when the condition occurs in other sites which include the ovaries, the utero-sacral ligaments, the rectovaginal septum, the pelvic peritoneum, the lower genital tract, the umbilicus, laparotomy scars, bowel, bladder and lymph nodes.

Aetiology

Endometriosis has been described as an enigmatic disease; its cause has certainly been the subject of much speculation and no one theory explains all cases. The endocrine background is uncertain, but it seems that the aberrant endometrium is hormone dependent. Oestrogen is presumed to be essential as the disease does not occur before the menarche and regresses after the menopause. It also regresses during pregnancy when much oestrogen is produced but this effect is probably the result of suppression of menstruation.

The main theories of the histogenesis of endometriosis are as follows:

1. *Direct implantation* would seem to be the most likely explanation for adenomyosis. The basal endometrium extends downwards into the myometrium and this continuity can sometimes be shown by serial histological section.
2. *Transplantation or 'retrograde menstruation'* probably accounts for most cases of ovarian or pelvic endometriosis. Tubal regurgitation of menstrual blood allows endometrial cells to implant on the ovary or peritoneum. The cells may not always implant directly; it may be that they contain an inductor substance which stimulates imitative metaplasia in susceptible tissues, for it has been shown experimentally that endometrium enclosed in a

millipore filter can induce endometriosis in adjacent tissues.

3. *Coelomic metaplasia.* The whole genital tract mucosa is derived from the coelomic epithelium, the primitive peritoneum. It seems possible therefore that endometriosis could result from abnormal differentiation of primitive cells. This would account for endometriosis in remote sites such as the umbilicus but on the whole it seems a less likely explanation for most cases than the transplantation theory.

4. *Lymphatic spread* may sometimes occur and may be responsible for the finding of endometriosis in lymph nodes, but no-one believes that this is a common cause of endometriosis.

5. *Blood spread* may explain some rare cases of endometriosis in limbs, lung and other unlikely sites.

Pathology

Adenomyosis usually causes symmetrical uterine enlargement but sometimes there may be localised lesions like fibroids but not encapsulated. On incising the myometrium pale areas with blood, spots are seen and histology shows these to contain endometrium. The characteristic of early pelvic endometriosis is the presence of small purple spots of aberrant endometrium at any point in the pelvic peritoneum, often in the region of the uterosacral ligaments and the pouch of Douglas. Endometriosis in the ovaries results in the formation of 'chocolate cysts', the chocolate coloured material being dark altered blood from which much fluid has been reabsorbed. (Such cysts may also be found in cases of haemorrhage from a corpus luteum). Chocolate cysts, even when quite small, may be associated with extensive adhesions, for the effusion of blood from any endometriotic tissue irritates the peritoneum with production of a fibrotic reaction and adhesions. In a severe case there may be a retroverted uterus involved in dense adhesions with endometrial extension into the rectosigmoid or posterior vaginal wall; one or both ovaries may be converted into large cysts (seldom, however, bigger than a grapefruit) which are adherent to the peritoneum of the pouch of Douglas and to bowel.

Microscopy may show endometrial glands and stroma in the affected tissues together with evidence of haemorrhage. In pregnancy the aberrant endometrium shows a decidual reaction. However, in about one third of all cases of extensive typical clinical endometriosis there is no histological evidence of the disease because of the destruction of the endometrial elements by pressure atrophy caused by haemorrhage. The term *endometrioid carcinoma* is used to describe cases of ovarian carcinoma where there is, in addition to obvious carcinoma, histological evidence of benign endometriosis and of a transition zone between benign and malignant tissue. The prognosis for endometrioid carcinoma is said to be better than that for carcinoma of the ovary in general. *Stromal endometriosis or adenomyosis* is a rare condition where endometrial stroma without glands invades the myometrium. This is usually benign but may sometimes act like a form of sarcoma.

Clinical features
Adenomyosis occurs typically in parous women between the ages of 40 and 50 and causes menorrhagia and dysmenorrhea. The uterus is enlarged and may be irregular and tender. The clinical features may not be distinguished from those of fibroids. Most patients with pelvic or ovarian endometriosis are younger, usually between 30 and 40 years; typically they are either nulliparous or relatively infertile and tend to belong to the higher social classes, including well educated women with responsible professional jobs. Occasionally endometriosis is found in teenage girls. Some gynaecologists have reported that endometriosis is increasing while others find a decrease in cases since the widespread use of oral contraception; it is difficult to get reliable figures. The most characteristic symptom of endometriosis is secondary dysmenorrhea which often includes backache and rectal pain if there is involvement of the utero-sacral ligaments and adjacent tissues. Dyspareunia may be severe. There is a high incidence of infertility although the tubes remain patent. Menstrual irregularities are common. It is one of the paradoxes of this disease that symptoms cannot be correlated with extent of the physical findings; extensive endometriosis will sometimes produce little discomfort while patients with minimal physical signs may have severe and incapacitating pain.

Diagnosis
The typical findings on examination of a patient with pelvic endometriosis are nodular thickening of the utero-sacral ligaments, fixed retroversion of the uterus and bilateral cystic ovaries. These features are of course very variable depending on the extent of the disease. It may be difficult to differentiate signs of endometriosis from those of chronic pelvic inflammatory disease. If large masses are present *laparotomy* should be performed as in any case of undiagnosed pelvic tumour.

Lesser degrees of endometriosis are diagnosed by *laparoscopy* and it may be useful to apply diathermy (carefully) to isolated small deposits, provided the bowel is well clear. Endometriosis involving the bowel itself may present the general surgeon with a problem for it can cause partial intestinal obstruction and may be difficult to differentiate from carcinoma of the colon or rectum.

Medical treatment

As has been stated there is no doubt that patients with substantial pelvic masses should have a laparotomy but in lesser cases of endometriosis the question of medical treatment arises. Endometriosis regresses during pregnancy and the administration of progestogens can produce clinical and histological improvement by inducing a decidual reaction in the endometrium.

If progestogens or oestrogen/progestogen combinations are given continuously so that amenorrhea is produced there may be considerable clinical improvement while the treatment is continued, but this is not universal. Cyclical treatment is less effective than continuous treatment. It is possible that the rather disappointing long-term results of oestrogen and progestogen treatment are because of the inherent stimulatory effects these hormones have on the endometrium. The ideal drug would be one which could induce atrophy of the endometrium without having any oestrogenic or progestational actions of its own. Danazol is a synthetic derivative of ethisterone which meets some of these requirements. It is said to have an antigonadotrophic action. 800 mg of danazol taken daily for 6 to 8 weeks will produce atrophy of the endometrium. Continuing the treatment for a number of months may alleviate the symptoms and signs of endometriosis and improvement has been confirmed by laparoscopy. Treatment with danazol may be valuable in patients with endometriosis who complain of infertility, for a pregnancy rate of 40 per cent after treatment has been reported. However, some patients may have recurrence of symptoms and signs after stopping danazol and surgery may be necessary. Danazol is much more expensive than progestogen preparations. Medical treatment is indicated for women with endometriosis who wish to have further children and women with minimal, incompletely removed or recurrent disease, but it does not replace surgery as a definitive treatment, nor does it avoid the need for diagnostic laparoscopy.

Surgical treatment

When endometriosis is extensive with bilateral cysts and widespread peritoneal deposits and particularly in older women, total hysterectomy and bilateral salpingo-oorphorectomy is the best treatment. In young women with less extensive disease, it is possible to remove the uterus and leave at least one ovary because hysterectomy itself will relieve the symptoms; the argument for such a procedure is less valid now that reliable hormone replacement therapy is available; oestrogen replacement after oophorectomy does not reactivate endometriosis.

Commonly, young women with endometriosis do not want a hysterectomy and an attempt at conservative surgery must then be made. This may involve resection of ovarian cysts, ventrisuspension of the uterus, diathermy to pelvic implants and similar procedures and may also be followed by a course of medical treatment.

If pregnancy follows, the disease may be cured permanently in some women.

There are others in whom there is a recurrence of disease after conservative surgery and, if a second operation is necessary, it should be radical.

FIBROIDS

Fibroids or myomata of the uterus are the commonest tumour in the human body. It is said that one in five women over the age of 35 has fibroids, although these are often small and cause no symptoms. The diagnosis and treatment of fibroids are often simple and straightforward but occasionally there are great difficulties which call for considerable surgical skill.

Aetiology

The cause of fibroids is unknown. They appear to arise from smooth muscle cells for small tumours consist purely of muscle fibres although large tumours also contain fibrous tissue. Fibroids form during reproductive life and never develop for the first time after the menopause. They tend to become larger during pregnancy and sometimes also in patients who are taking the contraceptive pill. It has been suggested that fibroids are the result of an abnormal response to oestrogens but there is no substantial evidence to prove this and it is difficult to understand why such a response should be localised to certain parts of the uterine muscle.

In European women fibroids are most commonly found over the age of 30 and often in nulliparous or relatively infertile women. In Negro women fibroids are very common at a younger age and despite normal fertility. The reason for this racial difference is also unknown.

Pathology

General features

Fibroids are usually multiple. Seedling fibroids first appear in the substance of the uterine muscle and compress the surrounding tissue to form a capsule. The presence of this capsule, from which the tumour can be enucleated is a characteristic feature and differentiates the fibromyoma from the adenomyoma which has no capsule.

Fibroids are gradually extruded from their original intramural or interstitial position either towards the uterine cavity where they become submucous (i.e. sub-endometrial) or towards the outer surface of the uterus where they become subserous (i.e. subperitoneal). Both submucous and subserous fibroids can become pedunculated. If a fibroid extends laterally between the leaves of the broad ligament, it is described as intraligamentary. Fibroids are said to occur 15 times more often in the body of the uterus than in the cervix, but cervical fibroids can sometimes attain great size so that the uterus may be pushed up on top of the tumour 'like the lantern on the dome of St. Paul's'. Fibroids in any position may vary extremely in size, from seedlings the size of a pin's head to vast tumours filling the abdomen and they frequently distort or displace the uterus with consequent difficulty in recognising normal anatomical landmards at operation. Great hypertrophy of the uterine vessels occurs to supply blood to the enlarged uterus but the tumours tend to outgrow their blood supply and this results in the well known degenerative changes.

Degenerative changes

Atrophy of most fibroids occurs after the menopause.

Hyaline degeneration is found in most large fibroids. Areas of the tumour become acellular with a pinkish amorphous appearance.

Cystic degeneration is a consequence of hyaline change; as hyalinisation increases there is a tendency towards liquefaction in the centre of the tumour.

Calcareous degeneration is common in large fibroids in older women and X-ray reveals multiple calcium deposits.

Red degeneration or necrobiosis is caused by an acute interference with blood supply – a form of infarction – and is usually seen during pregnancy. The tumour swells, softens and becomes red in colour. Necrobiosis is defined as a change in the direction of necrosis but with the tissues retaining the power of recovery.

Malignant degeneration in the form of sarcoma is rare in fibroids

– less than 0·5 per cent – but as fibroids are very common this is the most frequently found type of uterine sarcoma. It is usually unsuspected before operation. If the malignant change is confined within the fibroid, the prognosis may be favourable in comparison with other types of uterine sarcoma.

Other secondary changes

Torsion of a pedunculated fibroid may occur acutely, producing pain shock and vomiting but may sometimes pass undiagnosed. The tumour may become necrotic or may develop a blood supply from omental adhesions, becoming 'parasitic'.

Infection of a fibroid may occur after torsion and may sometimes be seen in necrotic submucous fibroid polyps which may extrude into the vagina as a sloughing mass.

Impaction of a fibroid in the pelvis may occur during menstruation or pregnancy and can produce acute retention of urine.

Clinical features

Symptoms. Symptoms of fibroids are extremely variable. Some large tumours may be completely asymptomatic while some small ones may cause considerable distress to the patient.

Menorrhagia is the commonest symptom and is usually associated with small or only moderately sized tumours; it is caused by enlargement of the endometrial surface, associated endometrial hyperplasia or by interference with uterine contractions. Profuse bleeding may cause severe anaemia and this is liable to occur in the case of a submucous fibroid which has escaped diagnosis at examination under anaesthesia and curettage.

Postmenopausal bleeding is not caused by fibroids, unless in the case of a fibroid polyp in the vagina or in the event of sarcomatous change. Neither do fibroids cause amenorrhea and if this occurs an associated pregnancy should always be suspected. Some patients with fibroids come with a complaint of abdominal swelling or with a history that an abdominal mass has been noted during routine examination for some other reason. It is remarkable that women may carry about tumours of great weight and size for many years without complaint.

Pressure on vessels may cause leg oedema, varicose veins or haemorrhoids. Pressure on the bladder may cause increased frequency of micturition or, occasionally, stress incontinence. Retention of urine may be cause by impaction of fibroids in the pelvis in the same way as by the retroverted gravid uterus. Infertility is associated with fibroids but is not produced by them;

fibroids are likely to develop in women who are infertile (either voluntarily or involuntarily) over a number of years.

Once fibroids have developed, in the late thirties or early forties, fertility has already decreased.

Signs. Fibroids can produce a variety of physical signs depending on their size, number, situation and the presence of secondary changes. Large fibroids are felt on abdominal examination as firm or hard, rounded, smooth, occasionally lobulated swellings arising out of the pelvis: on pelvic examination the whole mass is found to be continuous with the cervix and moves with it. Small fibroids within the pelvis are felt as firm or hard masses attached to the uterus which is asymmetrical, but a single intramural fibroid can cause symmetrical enlargement of the uterus.

Pedunculated fibroids may simulate solid ovarian tumours and vice versa.

The presence of fibroids should not obscure the clinician's mind to the possibility of other conditions, particularly pregnancy and ovarian carcinoma. Ascites is common in patients with ovarian carcinoma and uncommon in patients with fibroids.

Diagnosis

Because of the variability of clinical signs and symptoms, diagnosis can sometimes be difficult and in some cases is made only at laparotomy. If the abdominal mass is bigger than a 16 weeks pregnancy, laparotomy is usually advisable in any case. Laparoscopy has little place in the diagnosis of fibroids. When the fibroids are small the diagnosis may be settled by pelvic examination under anaesthesia and the passage of a uterine sound.

Ancillary diagnostic aids which are sometimes useful are X-ray and ultrasonic examination.

X-ray. A plain film of the abdomen can sometimes be very useful by detecting calcification. This degenerative change occurs in elderly women who are sometimes rather unfit for surgery. If calcification can be seen it can be assumed that the tumour mass is a fibroid and operation can sometimes be avoided. If no calcification is present the possibility of a solid ovarian tumour is much more likely and laparotomy may be essential to make the diagnosis. The other X-ray examination which may reveal a fibroid is hysterosalpingography which may show distortion of the uterine cavity by a submucous tumour.

Sonar. Sonar can differentiate between solid and cystic masses because ultrasound passes straight through fluid with hardly any absorbtion or reflection while it is absorbed in solid tissue. This means that the posterior wall of a cyst can be clearly seen but that it is difficult to demonstrate the posterior wall of a large solid fibroid. Degenerative changes in fibroids may confuse this typical appearance. Fibroids should be seen to be attached to the uterus while it should be possible to identify an ovarian tumour separately from the uterus.

Sonar is particularly useful for patients in whom an adequate clinical examination is impossible and is valuable in defining fibroids during pregnancy.

However, in many cases the information obtained by sonar is not of great practical value because the presence of a large pelvic mass is an indication for laparotomy. A final diagnosis can only be made after operation and histological examination.

Fibroids and pregnancy

Fibroids usually enlarge during pregnancy either because of increased blood supply or hormone stimulation and they tend to shrink during the puerperium. Fibroids sometimes become flattened as the uterus grows and compresses them. Most fibroids are lifted out of the pelvis as pregnancy advances and therefore do not interfere with engagement of the fetal head and with labour.

Abortion is said to be more common in women with fibroids and this is probably true when submucous fibroids are present but pregnancy may continue undisturbed even in women who have multiple large tumours. If the woman attends for antenatal care in the early months of pregnancy, fibroids are usually easily diagnosed on bimanual pelvic examination. One of the many advantages of screening by sonar in early pregnancy is that the fibroids can be accurately outlined.

Red degeneration (necrobiosis) is the most important complication of fibroids in pregnancy. It is quite likely that the patient will be known to have fibroids before red degeneration arises but the onset of symptoms is often quite sudden. Fairly acute abdominal pain is felt, localised over the tumour; there may be vomiting and the temperature and pulse may be elevated. The characteristic feature on abdominal examination is tenderness over the tumour, which moves with the uterus if the patient is turned on her side. Sometimes there is guarding and rigidity and the question of appendicitis may arise; other differential diagnoses to be considered are pyelonephritis and torsion of or haemorrhage into an ovarian tumour. Once the diagnosis of red degeneration is established the correct treatment is conservative. With analgesia, bed rest and local heat to the abdomen the patient's general and local condition will improve within 24 hours; if not, the diagnosis requires to be reviewed.

Occasionally, fibroids arising from the cervix or lower half of the uterus may cause an unstable lie in late pregnancy and eventually obstruct labour. Such patients need to be delivered by caesarean section. The temptation to perform myomectomy at the same time should be resisted for it is a dangerous operation because of the risk of haemorrhage; the only fibroids which should be removed at the time of caesarean section are small pedunculated ones.

In the puerperium, infection degeneration and torsion of fibroids may occur. Infection and degeneration should be treated conservatively. Torsion may require an operation.

Treatment of fibroids

Many fibroids do not cause symptoms and do not need treatment. When the diagnosis is certain and when fibroids are small and symptomless, patients can be reassured but should be asked to come for re-examination at six monthly intervals.

If menorrhagia is the only symptom and the fibroids are small, diagnostic curettage may be all that is required, particularly if the woman is approaching the age of the menopause. It is probably advisable to proceed to operation in every case where the diagnosis is in doubt, in every case where the tumour is larger than the size of a 16 weeks pregnancy and in every case where troublesome symptoms can be reasonably attributed to fibroids. Two operations are possible – myomectomy or hysterectomy. Myomectomy is indicated for young patients as it is possible for successful pregnancy to occur after the operation. Victor Bonney, who developed the modern technique of myomectomy and was a passionate advocate of the procedure maintained that, since cure without deformity or loss of function is the highest ideal of surgery, myomectomy is a greater surgical achievement than hysterectomy. Yet there is no doubt that it is often the more difficult operation of the two, that extensive enucleations of fibroids are associated with considerable haemorrhage, that convalescence may be complicated by haematoma formation and eventually there may be a lot of adhesions between the intestine and the suture lines on the uterus. Recurrence of fibroids occurs quite frequently after myomectomy. Hysterectomy is usually easier, causes less blood loss and post-operative morbidity, avoids the risk of recurrence of fibroids and guarantees relief of the symptoms they have been causing. Hysterectomy is the operation of choice for women who do not wish more children.

14

Ovarian cysts

Malignant tumours of the ovary are discussed in the Chapter on gynaecological cancer and all that will be done here is to mention, briefly, some of the clinical features of simple ovarian cysts. These are either distension cysts or cystic neoplasms.

Distension cysts

1. *Follicular cysts.* These are usually single and small, seldom growing larger than 5 cm in diameter. Most follicular cysts arise from atretic follicles. They do not become malignant and in most cases have no clinical significance. The cyst wall is made of an incomplete layer of granulosa cells enclosed in the theca layers of the follicle. Small follicular cysts are often felt on pelvic examination and seen at laparoscopy. Most of them require no treatment. Follicular cysts are quite frequently seen in association with pelvic inflammatory disease.

2. *Lutein cysts.* The commonest of these is the corpus lutein cyst. This is a cyst usually less than 5 cm in diameter. It may be associated with amenorrhoea. Occasionally, haemorrhage occurs into it and a ruptured corpus lutein cyst may cause free bleeding into the peritoneal cavity and simulate an ectopic pregnancy.

Theca-lutein cysts are the result of luteinisation of the granulosa and theca interna cells which line a follicular cyst. Bilateral multilocular theca lutein cysts occur in association with hydatidiform mole because of the excessive output of chorionic gonadotrophins. A similar change can be caused by drugs given to induce ovulation.

Cystic neoplasms

Mucinous cystadenoma. This is the commonest ovarian neoplasm. It may reach an enormous size, filling the whole abdomen. It contains multiple loculi, full of mucus. These loculi have a lining of tall columnar cells with nuclei close to the basement membrane and are separated by fibrous septa. If a mucinous cyst ruptures, the rare condition of myxoma peritonei may arise. Masses of mucin then collect in the peritoneal cavity and recur repeatedly after operative removal. This condition is probably due to dissemination of tumour cells. Although mucinous cysts of the ovary are so common, their origin is uncertain. They may be a kind of teratoma.

Serous cystadenoma. This may occur in either a simple or papilliferous form. Serous cysts seldom exceed 15 cm in diameter.

Endometrial cysts have already been discussed in the chapter on endometriosis.

Dermoid cysts. The dermoid cyst is a simple cystic teratoma which is most commonly found in young women of reproductive age. The cysts are enclosed in a firm fibrous capsule and contain yellow sebaceous material and a great variety of tissues, principally skin, hairs and teeth, but often including other elements such as bone, thyroid and gut. Dermoid cysts because of their weight, tend to lie in front of the uterus and as they are frequently on a long pedicle they are liable to torsion.

Clinical features

Symptoms. Ovarian cysts are often symptomless and, as with fibroids, they may attain great size before the patient comes to see the doctor. Large cysts eventually cause abdominal discomfort but pain is not a feature of smaller tumours unless complications such as torsion occur.

Signs. Typically a cystic, mobile, painless tumour can be felt separately from the uterus which is nearly always in front of it. Most large cysts come to occupy the midline in the abdomen and are smoothly rounded. Simple ovarian tumours are mobile unless they are very large. Dullness to percussion is elicited over the surface of the tumour and there is resonance in the flanks unless ascites is also present. Sonar examination can show ovarian cysts very clearly and should always be employed when there is doubt about the nature of an abdominal mass.

Ovarian cysts may easily be confused with the pregnant uterus and the use of sonar should eliminate this mistake.

Complications of ovarian cysts

Torsion

Torsion is liable to occur when the tumour is of moderate size and has a long pedicle. Small tumours can twist and untwist freely while large tumours do not have room to turn. When the pedicle twists the veins in it become obstructed and then the tumour becomes bereft of its blood supply and infarction occurs. This may be followed by necrosis and secondary infection. The typical symptoms are of recurrent abdominal pain and vomiting. The patient presents as an acute emergency and the finding of a tender cystic mass makes the diagnosis likely.

Rupture
Rupture of a cyst may follow a history of injury but sometimes it occurs spontaneously. There may be abdominal pain at the time of rupture and free fluid may be detected in the abdominal cavity. As has been stated, myxoma peritonei is the result of rupture of a mucinous cyst.

Infection
Infection of a cyst may occur in association with pelvic inflammatory disease or after torsion or in the puerperium. The cyst then becomes an abscess.

Incarceration
Incarceration of an ovarian cyst in the pelvis causes urinary retention.

Ovarian cysts and pregnancy
It is sometimes very difficult to diagnose ovarian cysts in association with pregnancy. Examination by sonar visualises them easily and should always be performed (if not routinely done in every antenatal patient) where there is clinical suspicion. Complications, such as torsion, rupture, incarceration or infection are more liable to occur in ovarian cysts in pregnancy. When ovarian tumours are diagnosed during pregnancy, they should be removed although it may be reasonable to wait until the first 12 weeks have passed so that the risk of abortion can be reduced. If the tumour is diagnosed for the first time during the last 4 weeks of pregnancy, removal of the cyst should be combined with Caesarean section.

Treatment of ovarian cysts
All ovarian cysts larger than 5 cm in diameter should be removed as soon as possible because of the risk of malignancy. Benign cysts can be resected by conservative cystectomy, leaving part of the ovary behind. This is particularly important in young women. In the patient who is approaching the age of the menopause, the correct treatment is bilateral salpingo-oophorectomy combined with total hysterectomy. All the tissues can then be subjected to complete histological examination and the presence or absence of

malignancy confirmed. When operating for ovarian cysts, every attempt should be made to remove them entirely. This may involve a large incision but the old practice of tapping followed by extraction of the collapsed cyst through a small incision is inadvisable because of the risk of the dissemination of malignant or myxomatous cells.

15

Gynaecological cancer

The diagnosis and treatment of malignant disease occupies a large part of the gynaecologist's time and efforts.

In our own gynaecological wards about a quarter of the patients are receiving treatment for cancer and the number of women investigated in the department as outpatients or attending for review is very considerable. Cancer of the uterus (including the cervix) and the ovaries when put together come second only to breast cancer in the list of new cases of malignant disease in women. Much effort has been put into gynaecological cancer research but there have been no great changes in reported cure rates except as a result of early diagnosis. The recovery of pre-malignant conditions has stressed the value of early detection and it is realised that excellent results can often be obtained if cancer is treated in its early stages. The public waits anxiously for the 'cure of cancer' as ancient peoples did for a sign from heaven. What it needed is education of both doctors and patients to use the facilities available to the full so that the significance of warning symptoms and signs is appreciated and treatment can be started promptly. Only an informed attitude on the part of the public will make new developments worthwhile.

CARCINOMA OF THE VULVA

This is a rare disease but it is of great interest to the gynaecological surgeon because it is the one form of genital malignancy in which radical surgery alone is clearly superior to every other kind of treatment. Vulvar cancer accounts for 3 to 4 per cent of all primary malignant tumours of the genital tract.

The average gynaecologist (if there is such a person) may see one or two cases each year. Stanley Way of Newcastle, who has a special experience of this disease, recorded seeing 642 cases in 34 years, an average of less than 20 a year. In view of its rarity, Way maintains that cancer of the vulva should always be treated in special centres which produce much better results than those obtained by individual surgeons.

Aetiology

The vulva provides conditions likely to lead to skin disturbance – warmth and moisture which are ideal for bacteria and friction from clothing which traumatises the epithelial surface. To these can be added the effects of poor hygiene and of scratching. The pathology of chronic skin conditions of the vulva is poorly understood. Jeffcoate's introduction of the term 'chronic vulval dystrophy' and abandonment of such traditional diagnosis as leukoplakia and kraurosis has helped to simplify nomenclature but basic knowledge of the causes awaits elucidation. Chronic vulvar skin changes may be degenerative, inflammatory or dysplastic and to make any diagnosis at all a biopsy is essential. Multiple small biopsies can be taken, using an instrument such as the Kilner hook, and any parts of skin which show induration or fissuring should always be sampled. Probably three small specimens should be taken from each side in most cases.

Clinical features

Cancer of the vulva is a disease of elderly women. Most cases occur between the ages of 50 and 70, although I have seen patients aged 29 and 89 years. There is usually a long history of pruritus vulvae but the woman's presenting symptom may seem comparatively trivial – 'soreness' of the vulva rather than pain, or some increase in itch, or a lump in the vulva. Delay in diagnosis is still common and this is mostly the patient's fault. Elderly women are often reluctant to come to the doctor with such complaints. Sometimes they treat themselves with ointments and sometimes, when they do attend the doctor, he does not examine them but merely gives them another prescription. All women complaining of pruritus vulvae should be examined locally in a good light, separating the labia to make sure that no cancer is hidden behind skin folds as it sometimes may be. Any lump or ulcer of the vulva should be subjected to biopsy at the earliest possible opportunity.

Cancer of the vulva is usually a typical epitheliomatous ulcer, but sometimes assumes a hypertrophic or 'cauliflower' form. It is usually situated on the anterior half of the vulva and affects mainly the skin of the labia majora. The surrounding skin may show evidence of an underlying vulval dystrophy. Inguinal glands may be palpable but the fact that they are not palpable does not mean that they are unaffected by growth.

Pathology
Most vulvar cancers are well-differentiated squamous carcinomata which, on histology, show typical epithelial pearl formation. Other tumours are undifferentiated with coalescent sheets of pleomorphic cells, some of which are multinucleated. The degree of anaplasia of the primary tumour has a vital bearing on the extent of lymph node involvement. Anaplastic tumours spread much more readily to deep lymph nodes and are therefore associated with a much worse prognosis than well-differentiated tumours.

The spread of vulvar cancer is by lymphatics and an understanding of the lymph drainage of the vulva is essential as a basis for treatment.

The lymphatics of the vulva lie mainly along the labia majora and do not spread laterally on to the thighs. The lymphatics on the medial surfaces of the labia minora flow forwards towards the vestibule.

Contralateral spread may occur between the lymphatics of the right and left sides of the vulva. Most of the lymphatics of the vulva drain directly to the superficial inguinal nodes and thence to the gland of Cloquet in the femoral canal.

Some lymph vessels from the clitoris drain directly to the gland of Cloquet.

There are five groups of lymph nodes arranged in two layers –

Superficial $\begin{cases} \text{Medial and lateral inguinal} \\ \text{Medial and lateral femoral} \end{cases}$

Deep $\begin{cases} \text{Inguinal} \\ \text{Femoral (including Cloquet's gland)} \\ \text{External iliac} \end{cases}$

The superficial and deep nodes have communications between them and all drain into the gland of Cloquet which is thus very important because it receives all the lymph drainage of the vulva.

This, at least, is the traditional teaching.

Way, however, maintains that the importance of the gland of Cloquet has been greatly over-rated and that this structure is seldom found at operation.

Management
Management begins with biopsy of any suspicious skin area on the vulva.

If the histological diagnosis is benign medical treatment may be applied and the patient kept under review. If carcinoma-*in-situ* (which may sometimes show the features of Bowen's or Paget's disease) is found, a simple vulvectomy is indicated, for the disease is often multicentric.

Where a clinical cancer of the vulva is present the biopsy should be taken from the growing edge of the tumour so that a true idea of its nature and of the degree of anaplasia can be obtained. Pieces taken from the middle of an ulcer are unsuitable for histology.

Having made the diagnosis of invasive cancer of the vulva, plans should be made for a radical vulvectomy. This operation should be carried out by the most experienced surgical team available.

Radical vulvectomy (first suggested by Basset in 1912 and popularised in Britain by Way since 1948) consists of excision of the vulva with bilateral superficial and deep lymphadenectomy. The incision removes a wedge of skin overlying the inguinal nodes in continuity with the vulva and its tumour.

It is important that removal of the vulva itself should be radical to avoid local recurrence which is always the danger after inadequate surgery.

It is the usual practice to submit the nodes when they are excised during the operation to the pathologist for immediate frozen section. If the inguinal nodes are clear, further extension of the operation can be avoided. If the deep nodes are affected it may be necessary to divide the inguinal ligament and dissect out the internal iliac nodes. This is a comparatively rare event in my small experience. On conclusion of the dissection and after securing as much haemostasis as possible an attempt should be made to close the skin edges. The groin wounds are closed with continuous suction drainage and the vulvar wound is closed without drainage. Local sepsis may be reduced by using an antibiotic spray during the operation.

It is surprising how well the patients (even frail and elderly women) tolerate this operation (provided the inguinal ligament is not divided) and how little post-operative discomfort they have. They should be encouraged to get up early and if the skin incisions heal well they can go home in three or four weeks. The overall five year survival from radical vulvectomy in the best hands is 70 per cent. When the deep nodes are involved, however, the survival rate is only 33 per cent.

The operation is worthwhile in practically every case for it will save the patient a miserable death from a foul fungating painful growth.

Other vulvar tumours

For a discussion on rarer tumours such as basal-cell carcinoma, melanoma, carcinoma of Bartholin's gland and carcinoma of the urethra, the reader is referred to a textbook of gynaecological pathology (see list of suggestions for further reading).

CARCINOMA OF THE VAGINA

This is an even rarer disease than cancer of the vulva for all types of vaginal cancer together account for only 1 to 2 per cent of all genital tract malignancies. Treatment is difficult and the prognosis is poor. Secondary cancer of the vagina is commoner than primary.

Carcinoma-in-situ of the vagina

Carcinoma-*in-situ* of the vagina is probably part of a multicentric process, the most common association being with carcinoma-*in-situ* of the cervix. It may occur after hysterectomy for cervical carcinoma-*in-situ* and I have seen such a case, where the vaginal lesion at first showed intra-epithelial changes only and later became an invasive carcinoma. The patient was then treated with radiotherapy.

Primary invasive epidermoid carcinoma of the vagina

This accounts for less than 0·5 per cent of genital malignancies. Its commonest site is on the posterior vaginal wall and it may spread to involve the rectum. Lymphatic extension is similar to that seen in cervical cancer.

Cases should be classified as primary carcinoma of the vagina only when the site of growth is clearly in the vagina only.

A growth that involves the cervix should be classifed as carcinoma of the cervix. A growth that has extended to the vulva should be classified as carcinoma of the vulva. A growth that is limited to the urethra should be classified as carcinoma of the urethra.

Primary carcinoma of the vagina is usually of squamous type and is found mostly in post-menopausal women. The only aetiological factor of note is the wearing of a pessary, which if retained for years may cause ulceration and cancer.

Clear-celled adenocarcinoma of the vagina

This is of particular interest because it is an example of cancer caused by an agent acting during fetal life. In the U.S.A. in

1970–71 eight cases of this extremely rare disease were found among adolescent girls and investigation showed that seven of the eight mothers had been treated with stilboestrol during the first three months of the pregnancy from which the girls were born. Many more cases have been reported since then, but there have been none in Britain. These adenocarcinomas seem related to pre-existing vaginal adenosis and it has been found that some girls exposed to stilboestrol in fetal life who did not have adeno-carcinomas did have adenosis.

Secondary carcinoma of the vagina
This may arise from a primary in the uterus (notably after hyster-ectomy for endometrial carcinoma) from the vulva, ovary, kidney, bladder, urethra, bowel or from choriocarcinoma. Vaginal second-aries from endometrial carcinoma may be prevented by removing a cuff of vagina at the time of operation and by post-operative irradiation of the vagina.

Treatment of vaginal carcinoma
Treatment of vaginal carcinoma may pose a difficult problem because of the proximity of bladder and rectum and varies accord-ing to the origin of the tumour. Squamous tumours are probably best treated with radiotherapy, choriocarcinoma responds to chemotherapy while areas of carcinoma-*in-situ* may respond to local ablation under colposcopic direction. Surgery, in the form of complete vaginectomy, is a formidable procedure and there are few who have experience of it, but this is the treatment which was employed for many of the young American girls with clear-celled adenocarcinoma.

CARCINOMA OF THE CERVIX

The cervix is easily accessible to diagnostic techniques; early diag-nosis of cancer of the cervix allows treatment which is almost certain to cure the disease. Even in its invasive form, cancer of the cervix is associated with characteristic symptoms and signs which have been taught to medical students for generations and, there-fore, referral for treatment while the chance of cure remains good should often be possible. Nevertheless, cancer of the cervix remains the cause of a substantial number of deaths, particularly among middle-aged women. It causes about 2200 deaths each year in England and Wales and about half these deaths occur in women aged between 45 and 64 years.

Aetiology
Aetiological factors have been studied extensively and some of the main ones are as follows.

1. *Social.* Death rates from cancer of the cervix vary according to marital status and social class. The death rate in single women is half the rate in married women, which, in turn, is half the rate in divorced women. The death rate in social class V is about 5 times the death rate in social class I. About two fifths of the deaths from cancer of the cervix in women over the age of 35 occur in social classes IV and V.

The association between cancer of the cervix and early coitus, frequent coitus, promiscuity, failure to use occlusive contraceptives and similar factors is well known. The 'high-risk groups' for venereal disease also have a high risk of developing cancer.

2. *Infections.* In addition to the association with venereal disease, smegma has been incriminated as an infective agent although evidence is indefinite. Another male factor of importance is semen which may be an ideal medium for the replication of carcinogenic viruses. The most important of these is Herpes virus Type 2 (HSV-2). HSV-2 is transmitted by sexual intercourse and the epidemiological features of HSV-2 infection and cervical cancer are similar. Infectious HSV-2 has been found on cells cultured from carcinoma-*in-situ*.

HSV-2 is carcinogenic in animals.

HSV-2 antigen has been found in cells from carcinoma of the cervix and antibodies to HSV-2 are increased in women with invasive and pre-invasive carcinoma of cervix as compared with controls.

3. *Immunological factors.* Both intra-epithelial and invasive carcinoma of the cervix are more common in women who are immuno-suppressed than in the general population. The reasons for this are not yet clear.

4. *The contraceptive pill.* Not surprisingly this has attracted publicity as a possible cause of cancer. There is no direct link and cancer of the cervix is just as preventable in those who use the pill as in those who do not.

Pathology
The morbid anatomy of the disease and its mode of spread are well summarised by the classification adopted by the International Federation of Obstetrics and Gynaecology (FIGO). Stages 0 and Ia comprise pre-clinical carcinoma, diagnosed by cytology, colpo-

scopy and histology. The other stages are based on clinical examination when the patient first presents: this usually means the pelvic examination made under general anaesthesia when biopsy is taken.

Stage 0:   Intra-epithelial carcinoma (carcinoma-*in-situ*).

Stage Ia: { Intra-epithelial carcinoma with micro-invasion.
            { Occult invasive carcinoma.

Stage Ib: Frankly invasive carcinoma confined to the cervix.

Stage II: Invasive carcinoma which extends beyond the cervix but has not reached the lateral pelvic wall or lower third of vagina.

Stage III: Invasive carcinoma which extends to either lateral pelvic wall and/or lower third of vagina.

Stage IV: Invasive carcinoma which involves the urinary bladder, rectum or extends beyond the true pelvis.

The distinction between micro-invasive carcinoma and occult invasive carcinoma is difficult to make and there is no uniform definition. Some gynaecologists think that the whole concept of 'micro-invasion' should be abandoned: this diagnosis, they maintain, merely lets the pathologist off the hook and transfers responsibility to the clinician who requires to treat the case either as one of carcinoma-*in-situ* or invasive carcinoma, the more correct treatment being probably the former.

The most important means of spread of cervical carcinoma is by direct invasion. Lymphatic spread occurs by embolisation but blood-borne metastases are late and comparatively rare. The ureters are affected by direct invasion or by compression in two thirds of patients and about half the deaths from cervical cancer are attributable to uraemia.

On *histological examination* the carcinoma infiltrates as a network of anastomosing bands which on section appear as irregular islands of malignant cells. Various attempts have been made to grade cancers according to their histological features. Well-differentiated cancers show circular whorls of cells with central nests of keratin: there are large hyperchromatic nuclei with coarse chromatin. In the moderately-differentiated group, keratin pearls are not seen and nuclear polymorphism is more obvious, while poorly-differentiated tumours consist of small round cells with dark nuclei and numerous mitotic figures.

95 per cent of cervical cancers are squamous growths: the remaining 5 per cent are adenocarcinomata which are the predominant type in very young patients.

Clinical features

Carcinoma-*in-situ* and micro-invasive carcinoma have no clinical features, the diagnosis being made by the microscope.

Once the tumour becomes invasive, abnormal bleeding occurs from broken vessels on its surface. This bleeding may be post-coital, inter-menstrual or post-menopausal. Such symptoms are of the utmost importance and demand immediate investigation. Any abnormal bleeding in women aged over 35 should be assumed to be caused by cancer until proved otherwise.

A foul discharge is a late symptom indicating ulceration and infection of the growth.

Pain indicates widespread involvement of nerves and occurs only when the tumour is far advanced. Uraemia may be revealed clinically and some patients may have fistulae into bladder or bowel causing incontinence.

On *clinical examination* of a woman with invasive cancer of the cervix, the gynaecologist will usually find the typical rough, friable indurated lesion, sometimes with extensive local ulceration. The growth tends to assume two main forms, the everting or exophytic variety which gives rise to the 'cauliflower' type of growth and the inverting or endophytic variety which results in ulceration and induration of the tissues of the cervix. Parametrial spread is best assessed by rectal examination and formal staging of the growth should be done on pelvic examination under anaesthesia when a biopsy can also be taken.

Screening for cervical cancer

The cervical smear test has been in use for more than 30 years. Despite its world-wide employment on a vast scale it is still uncertain whether this test helps to reduce mortality from cervical cancer.

In British Columbia, where a special effort has been made, a reduction in the morbidity and mortality from cervical carcinoma is claimed, but, even there, 20 per cent of the population have remained unscreened and in that 20 per cent are a large number of very young and of elderly women, of women of low social class who are urban dwellers – in other words a high proportion of those who are most at risk from the disease.

Other problems in assessing the results of screening programmes and their effect on mortality are that many of the lesions detected by cytology would have a good prognosis anyway, either because the lesion never became invasive or because of the efficiency of treatment for cancer in its early stages; also it is possible that some cancers develop so rapidly that they never go through the intra-epithelial stage at all and are never caught by any screening programme.

Any expansion of screening facilities should be directed to women who would not otherwise attend. Some form of domiciliary service may need to be devised. The greatest contribution the general practitioner can make to the cure of cervical cancer is to ensure that all his female patients attend in systematic fashion over a period of years and have their cervical smears taken either by him or at an appropriate clinic.

Cytology and the clinician

Taking a cervical smear requires skill and great emphasis should be placed on this when undergraduates are taught practical gynae-cology. Even for experienced gynaecologists, it is not always easy to get a clear view of the cervix or to take an adequate scrape from its surface. Yet thousands of smears are being taken by inexperi-enced people and decisions are being taken about patients on the basis of poor samples.

My own technique is to locate the cervix first by gentle pal-pation with one finger so that the speculum can be more easily and comfortably passed in the right direction. Such preliminary palpation of the cervix has been criticised as meddlesome because it may remove superficial cells before a smear can be taken. My answer is that the blind passage of the speculum can abrade the cervix much more easily than the finger. I have seen, through the colposcope, a whole sheet of superficial cells lifted off by the passage of the speculum. When the cervix is clearly seen the Ayres spatula should be rotated over its whole surface, paying particular attention to the squamo-columnar junction (the transformation zone of the colposcopists).

Cytologists usually grade smears something like this:

Grade I   Normal.
Grade II   Slight atypia (e.g. in metaplasia or infection).
Grade III   Dysplasia.
Grade IV   Dysplasia with cells suspicious of malignancy.
Grade V   Malignant cells with nuclear changes and basal dys-
            karyosis.

Communication between cytologist and clinician should be clear: personal contact by visit or telephone is best if there is any doubt-ful feature. The clinician's response to the cytology report is likely to be something like this:

Grade I   If normal – repeat smear in 2 years.

Grade II   If trichomonal infection, treat it and then repeat the smear.

Grade III ⎫

Grade IV ⎬ If there is any feature suggestive of cancer, a diagnosis should be made by colposcopy or biopsy.

Grade V   ⎭

Colposcopy

Colposcopy is usually employed as a second screening procedure for:

1. Those with abnormal smears.
2. Those with a clinically abnormal cervix.

Colposcopy is an out-patient procedure involving no discomfort for the patient provided she is treated with sympathy and sensitivity to her own feelings. The colposcope is a low power binocular microscope which gives a stereoscopic view of the cervix at magnification of × 6 to × 40. By using a green filter, contrast is increased, for red appears as black which makes examination of sub-epithelial capillaries easier.

The cervix is exposed with a bivalve speculum and mucus wiped away. Acetic acid 3 per cent is then applied to the cervix with a cotton wool swab. This causes columnar or abnormal epithelium to swell and makes it easier to recognise. The disadvantage of using acetic acid is that it disturbs the vascular pattern. The capillaries are best studied while keeping the cervix moist with normal saline. The transformation zone, frequently concentric with the os, is the most important area for colposcopic study for it is the main site of neoplastic transformation. The colposcope can define precisely the normal from the abnormal transformation zone; this distinction is made on the basis of colour and superficial blood vessel distribution. A mosaic structure of the epithelium and the presence of atypical vessels are among the changes that may be seen.

The object of colposcopy is to identify suspicious areas so that biopsy (which can be done during colposcopic examination) can provide tissue for histological diagnosis. When there is a discrepancy between the findings on colposcopy and histology it is usually the practice to accept the histological diagnosis as the correct one. However, the histological diagnosis should not be accepted uncritically for the histologist has many problems associated with the cutting and staining of the sections. Interpretation may vary with the experience and subjective judgment of the pathologist who shares with common humanity the capacity for error.

Treatment of patient with epithelial changes on her cervix
The basic definitions of epithelial change of the cervix are:

Dysplasia – basal layers showing some of the cytological changes of cancer but superficial layers showing some differentiation.

Carcinoma-*in-situ* – carcinomatous change throughout the whole thickness of the epithelium but no sub-epithelial invasion.

Hysterectomy. This seemed to many cutting gynaecologists the best treatment for a woman with a pre-malignant cervical lesion. 'Extended hysterectomy' (usually meaning the additional removal of a vaginal cuff) also became popular. If, however, the lesions were multicentric as sometimes happens, no amount of extension would eradicate disease. I have seen two patients with ureteric fistulae following extended hysterectomy for carcinoma-*in-situ*.

A great advance occurred when it was found that conisation of the cervix was therapeutic as well as diagnostic for carcinoma-*in-situ*. Hysterectomy for carcinoma-*in-situ* is now reserved for the following groups:

1. Those in whom another indication is present (e.g. fibroids, menorrhagia).
2. Those who show abnormal smears and colposcopy after conisation.
3. Those who have lesions in upper vagina – but beware of multicentric disease.

Conisation of the cervix. As definitive treatment for carcinoma-*in-situ* this has produced good results. A large cone biopsy is therapeutic in more than 90 per cent of cases.

When performing the operation haemostasis should be made as complete as possible but the Sturmdorf technique should not be used for covering the cervix as it may cover over residual pathological tissue.

A large cone biopsy, by any technique, carries with it a considerable risk of complications.

Secondary haemorrhage may be dramatic and profuse, pelvic infection may supervene and the end result may be a stenosed or incompetent cervix. There is an argument therefore for leaving as much normal tissue as possible, particularly in the child-bearing years.

Colposcopically directed cone biopsies tend to be smaller, have fewer complications and seem to be just as therapeutic as the more radical procedures.

Colposcopy has made intelligent conservatism possible.

Local excision of the lesion. This treatment which has extended conservatism even further but such treatment is for skilled coposcopists only. If the lesion can be localised by colposcopy, punch or wedge biopsy may remove it. After a histological diagnosis has been obtained from the punch biopsy localised destruction of remaining lesions may be done by the cryo-cautery, electro-diathermy or CO_2 laser.

Cryo-cautery. This painless out-patient procedure, is indicated for small superficial areas of dysplasia: destruction does not penetrate below 3 cm.

Electro-diathermy. Electro-diathermy under general anaesthesia is indicated if deeper penetration is desired. A histological diagnosis from a colposcopically directed biopsy is required. Electro-diathermy can destroy lesions to a depth of 1 cm.

The CO_2 laser. This can destroy very small areas of tissue with great precision to any required depth and can be used as an out-patient procedure. It may have a great future in association with colposcopy.

The patient who has persistent epithelial abnormality after treatment poses problems.

With colposcopy the residual lesion can often be identified and treated appropriately (whether by conisation, hysterectomy or otherwise).

If a positive smear shows up after hysterectomy, it may be possible to destroy or remove the lesions on the vagina depending on the colposcopic findings. Such treatment may avoid extensive radiation or dangerous radical operations like vaginectomy.

The investigation of patients with invasive cancer of the cervix
On admission the patient should have a general medical examination so that her fitness for any necessary treatment can be assessed. Blood is taken for a full blood count and relevant biochemical tests including urea and electrolytes.

A careful abdominal examination should be made during the admission procedure but as the patient has usually had a pelvic examination at the out-patient clinic, a repeat of this can often be deferred until the formal examination under anaesthetic is performed. An X-ray of chest and an intravenous pyelogram are best performed before the patient goes to theatre.

Examination under anaesthesia is of the greatest importance for this is the occasion on which the growth is staged and decisions about treatment made. It is preferable that both gynaecologist and the radiotherapist should be present to ensure close-co-operation in treatment. A careful bimanual examination should reveal the local extent of the cancer and, combined with rectal examination, the degree of parametrial infiltration. A biopsy of the cervix should be taken and if possible this should include some normal as well as malignant tissue so that the pathologist can give an opinion about the degree of invasion histologically. Sometimes all the accessible tissue is so friable that this is not possible and in these cases the best way is to break off a piece with the curette. Cystoscopy should be part of this initial examination of the patient: bullous oedema indicates spread to underlying bladder muscle and direct invasion of the bladder mucosa is present in about 2 per cent of cases.

When all the clinical information is assembled *staging* of the growth is done according to the FIGO classification. When in doubt, the earlier of two stages should always be chosen and under no circumstances must clinical staging be altered once treatment has started.

Once the initial staging and biopsy are done treatment can usually proceed without delay but there are a number of other investigations which are sometimes used for patients with cervical cancer and they can be conveniently mentioned at this point.

Lymphangiography. This procedure is more favoured by radiotherapists than gynaecologists. It is tedious and uncomfortable for the patient and may involve a risk of embolisation with tumour cells or fat. In any case the films are very difficult to read. Many gynaecologists feel that lymphangiography is of little practical help in the management of patients with cervical carcinoma.

Sonar. Sonar has been used to provide measurements from fixed points in the pelvis to act as a guide to radiotherapists in their treatment and is also of value in the diagnosis of local recurrence and spread of the tumour. The detection of a hydronephrosis or alteration in bladder contour may indicate spread to the urinary tract.

X-ray skeletal survey. This may be indicated in patients with extensive disease or recurrence although bone metastases from cervical carcinoma are comparatively rare.

Isotope scans. Isotope scans of bone and liver may also help to identify distant metastases, particularly in cases of recurrence.

Treatment of invasive cancer of the cervix
Since the early years of the twentieth century, when radical hysterectomy and radiotherapy both became practical possibilities, a debate has raged about which method is the best treatment for cervical cancer. At no time have there been any reports of controlled series in which patients have been randomly allocated to either radiotherapy or surgery. The argument between surgery and radiotherapy still goes on but it is a sterile and often childish one and it should cease.

The real factors which determine the method of treatment for any patient are:

1. The facilities available.
2. The needs of the individual woman and the extent of her disease.
3. The training and temperament of the gynaecologist, because radical surgery requires a bold extrovert whose skills are kept sharp by constant use.

The best results are obtained where a full oncological service is available, when gynaecologists, radiotherapists, pathologists and experts in cancer chemotherapy meet, talk to each other and plan joint projects.

Specialists in urology, renal medicine and other disciplines should also be available for consultation. In participating in such a scheme, the gynaecological surgeon needs to develop the Christian virtue of self-denial. Much as he might enjoy the occasional 'Wertheim', there is no place now for the occasional surgeon in the treatment of cancer of the cervix, except in regions where no other facilities exist.

World opinion favours radiotherapy as the treatment of choice for all stages of invasive cervical cancer, but in most countries there are some centres where surgery is preferred.

Surgery, as a primary treatment, is usually reserved for specially selected 'operable' cases. Radiotherapy is applicable to everyone and cases are unselected; it can be used for the obese, the elderly and patients who are poor medical risks. Complications of radiation have been much reduced since the introduction of supervoltage therapy. Surgery is essential when radiotherapy is not available, when the tumour is radio-resistant or when there is recurrence after complete radiation treatment.

Approximate five year survival rates from large series treated by radiotherapy are as follows:

Stage I: 75 per cent
Stage II: 55 per cent
Stage III: 30 per cent
Stage IV: 10 per cent

The overall five year survival rate for all stages is in the region of 50 per cent.

The principle of radiotherapy for cervical cancer is that the local tumour and its immediate paracervical spread is attacked with intrauterine and intravaginal sources of radiation while the pelvic lymphatics and nodes are dealt with mainly by external radiation.

The original techniques of radiotherapy were:

Stockholm: High intensity radiation of short duration was given 3 times in 3 weeks.
Paris: Low intensity radiation was given continuously for a period up to a week.
Manchester: Pre-determined doses delivered to fixed points within the pelvis, usually by two insertions with an interval of a week or 10 days between them.

Recently *Cesium-137* has tended to supplant radium. As a by-product of nuclear fission it is less expensive than radium. Another advantage is that it emits only γ-rays of uniform energy and penetrability. It is also safer for medical, nursing and technical staff, particularly if the 'after-loading' technique to be described is used.

Radiation is measured in rads. The rad is the absorbed dose of radiation which is accompanied by the liberation of 100 ergs of energy per gram of absorbing material.

The intensity of radiation varies inversely with the square of the distance between the point source of the energy and the point of its effect.

Dosage to the cervix and pelvic lymph nodes is related to two points on each side of the pelvis.

Point A: 2 cm lateral to axis of uterine canal and 2 cm above the vaginal fornix.
Point B: 3 cm lateral to point A.

It is usual to have two applications of Cesium-137 to the cervix supplemented by external treatment from the linear accelerator. The 'after loading' technique is as follows.

A tube is inserted into the uterus and avoids into the fornices. All these sources have tubes attached through which the radioactive material can be inserted. At the initial application 'dummies' can be inserted for taking dosimetry films. The vagina is packed to keep the sources of radiation in position and as well away from bladder and rectum as possible.

An X-ray confirms that the applicators are in proper position. When application is satisfactory the patient is taken to a protected area where the correct sources of cesium are put into each applicator. A scintillation counter then measures the amount of radiation being received by the rectum and checks that it is acceptable.

Two cesium applications are made at weekly intervals.

External irradiation by the 4 MV linear accelerator is then given in about 20 divided daily doses.

The combined treatment delivers about 8500 rads to point A and 5000 rads to point B.

Sometimes, external radiation is given first, e.g. to shrink bulky tumours and make the subsequent local insertion easier.

Variations in treatment may be adopted according to the stage of the tumour.

Stage Ia. Here, as has already been stated, the clinician's decision is whether to treat these cases of 'microinvasion' and 'occult invasion' as carcinoma-*in-situ* or invasive carcinoma. If the former, a large cone biopsy or simple hysterectomy will suffice; if the latter, many gynaecologists would opt for radiotherapy.

Stage Ib. In hands of experts there is little difference between the results of surgery and radiotherapy, but morbidity (particularly ureteric damage) is probably greater with surgery.

Stage II. Radiotherapy – either intracavity radiation followed by external radiation to the whole pelvis or sometimes external radiation followed by local application.

Stage III. Intracavity radiation may be useful initially to shrink the tumour or control haemorrhage. A large dose of external radiation is necessary to cope with the wide spread of the tumour so that the risk of complications of radiotherapy is greater. Radiation given in hyperbaric oxygen may be useful in some Stage III cases, the theory being that tumours are more radiosensitive if their oxygenation is increased; results show an improvement in the local clearance of the tumour but survival rates are disappointing.

Stage IV. Treatment is palliative. Radiation is haemostatic and may reduce pain and leg oedema.

Surgical operations for urinary or bowel diversion should be employed as indicated. In special circumstances, exenteration should be considered but only if it is thought that performing the operation will give the patient a better quality of life.

Follow-up of patients treated for cervical cancer
The follow-up should be life long. Patients should be seen every three months for the first two years, every six months for the next three years and annually thereafter. Questions should be asked about their general health and occupation so that an idea of their 'quality of life' is obtained. A blood sample should be taken to exclude anaemia. Abdominal, vaginal and rectal examination are done to detect any changes in the pelvis. Patients who have had radiotherapy always have marked parametrial induration and this is a normal finding. Taking a smear for cytology is of doubtful value as the results may be very confusing. X-rays and special investigations are ordered when indicated. Attendance at a cancer follow-up clinic is often a surprisingly cheerful and encouraging experience for patient and doctor alike and the atmosphere should be one of brisk optimism.

Management of recurrent cervical carcinoma
In contrast this is, however, a gloomy subject.

Of those women with recurrence after initial apparently adequate treatment only 15 per cent survive one year and only 5 per cent survive 5 years. Their management depends upon whether there seems to be a hope of cure or whether palliation is the only possible treatment. An attempt at cure may be made by radiation or surgery where there are isolated central pelvic recurrences or metastases in the lower vagina.

Radiation is sometimes very effective when the recurrence arises outside the previously treated area – e.g. a bone metastasis – and it can give relief of symptoms and local control of the tumour.

Patients with inoperable recurrence and intractable pain present difficult problems which tax the art of medicine to its limits.

The main rôle of exenteration seems to be in carefully selected cases of recurrent carcinoma. The risks of these formidable operations are great but some of the patients who survive seem to be able to lead remarkably normal lives.

Complications of radiotherapy
As has been stated complications are much fewer than in the past.
Leukopenia. This is seldom severe and the white cells do not fall to the low levels associated with the use of cytotoxic drugs.
Skin burns. These are now rarely seen, for the use of multiple

ports of entry, rotational methods and high voltage therapy have avoided the worst effects. Occasionally, slight erythema and subsequent pigmentation are encountered.

Vaginal stenosis. Vaginal stenosis of some degree is almost inevitable but is not untreatable. Oestrogen creams and coitus are the best methods of treatment.

Urinary symptoms. These include frequency and dysuria which may be caused by transient cystitis.

Telangiectasia of the bladder wall. This may cause haematuria.

Avascular necrosis of the bladder wall. This may lead to vesico-vaginal fistula which is not usually apparent until about 6 months after radiotherapy.

Obstruction of the ureters. The ureters are seldom damaged by treatment but may be later obstructed by radiation fibrosis of the surrounding tissues.

Gastro-intestinal symptoms. These are fairly common. Many patients have an entero-colitis with nausea, diarrhoea and generalised weakness. Spontaneous recovery is usual but the course of radiotherapy may need to be stopped temporarily. In some cases there may be a plastic peritonitis which causes adhesions and intestinal obstruction: this can often be treated conservatively by intravenous drip and gastric suction.

Future management of cancer of cervix

Future management may be affected by rapid developments in the field of cancer chemotherapy, but there has been little fundamental advance in the treatment of this disease for many years.

Perhaps the most practical step which clinicians can take is to improve schemes for early diagnosis and make a specific attempt to reach those women who are most at risk. If there were a will in the community to eradicate cervical cancer completely, it would be found that the way to do it is already available.

CARCINOMA OF THE ENDOMETRIUM

Tutorials on this subject often start off by contrasting endometrial carcinoma with carcinoma of the cervix, pointing out that it is an adeno carcinoma, not a squamous carcinoma; that it is within a closed muscular box, the uterus, rather than on a surface which is virtually external and is exposed to trauma and infection; that it spreads slowly and mainly by direct invasion, that the women it affects are of different age and parity from those with cancer of the cervix and that its primary treatment is surgery, not radiotherapy.

The prognosis is slightly more favourable than that of cervical carcinoma but there has been virtually no change in the cure rate for the past 20 years.

Incidence
Carcinoma of the endometrium used to be reported as 6 times less common than cervical carcinoma but this proportion is changing rapidly. In 1971 carcinoma of the endometrium was responsible for more than half the deaths from uterine cancer in England and Wales and in many places cancer of the endometrium is now just as common as cancer of the cervix. This may not be because of an absolute increase in endometrial cancer but rather because of a decrease in the number of cases of invasive cancer of the cervix.

Age
Cancer of the endometrium is usually found in post-menopausal women, its maximum incidence being at age 61. Three quarters of the patients are over the age of 50.

Parity
These patients are a relatively infertile group. Only about half of them have had children, so it could be said that cancer of the endometrium is equally common in parous and nulliparous women.

Previous menstrual history
Attempts have been made to relate cancer of the endometrium to previous menstrual abnormalities, influenced by the idea that overstimulation of the endometrium may lead to cancer. It has been said that half the women with endometrial carcinoma have had a history of menorrhagia and that women who menstruate after the age of 50 make up more than half the cases of endometrial carcinoma.

When the radium menopause was a popular treatment it was calculated that women who had this were three times more likely to develop endometrial carcinoma than expected – the cause of this association may have been the heavy bleeding for which the radium was originally given. In any case, the argument has little relevance now as menopausal radium is practically obsolete.

Obesity, hypertension and diabetes
These are general medical disorders which have been supposed to have a special relationship to endometrial carcinoma but the evidence for this is very doubtful. Every gynaecological surgeon

knows to his cost that many patients with endometrial carcinoma are fat, but so also are women of a similar age who have, for example, gall bladder disease.

It is probable that obesity, hypertension and diabetes do not occur more frequently among patients with endometrial carcinoma than in the general population of women of similar age.

Oestrogens
The relationship with oestrogens requires to be taken more seriously. The idea that endometrial carcinoma is an oestrogen dependent tumour is an old one and has received some recent support in that there is now strong circumstantial evidence that oestrogen replacement therapy, given for menopausal symptoms, is associated with endometrial carcinoma. It has also been shown that exogenous oestrogens in high dosage can cause uterine cancer in rabbits.

It is tempting to believe that endogenous oestrogens can also be carcinogenic and that the pathogenesis of endometrial carcinoma involves a transition from normal endometrium to cystic hyperplasia, then to atypical adenomatous hyperplasia, then to adeno-carcinoma. All these types of endometrium tend to merge into each other and it is sometimes very difficult even for pathologists of great experience to tell the difference between atypical endometrial hyperplasia and endometrial carcinoma. Sometimes hyperplastic and carcinomatous tissue are found adjacent on the same histological section. However, sections have also been shown where endometrial carcinoma can be seen adjacent to secretory endometrium and this rather upsets the theory.

The traditional endocrinological explanation of the genesis of endometrial carcinoma is that unopposed oestrogen stimulation is the main factor. Yet many patients with endometrial carcinoma are shown to have atrophic vaginitis (a clinical sign of oestrogen deficiency) and urinary oestrogen levels are not raised in post-menopausal women with endometrial carcinoma.

A complex interplay of endocrine factors is probably involved in these cases. It has recently been claimed that there is an increased conversion of the adrenal androgen, androstenedione, to oestrone in post-menopausal women with cystic hyperplasia of the endometrium and this mechanism may be of some aetiological importance in endometrial carcinoma, for oestrone is the predominant circulating oestrogen in some women with endometrial carcinoma.

Methods of early diagnosis of endometrial cancer

Any improvement in the prognosis of endometrial cancer must be associated with earlier detection of the disease and it would seem that this should involve more knowledge about its hormone dependency.

As has been shown, the link with oestrogens is complex but it would seem advisable as a prophylaxis against endometrial cancer, to stop unopposed continuous therapy with synthetic oestrogens and replace it with cyclical oestrogen/progesterone mixtures.

There has been a need for a screening test similar to exfoliative cytology for cervical carcinoma and various methods to devise one have included sponge biopsy of the endometrium, vacuum curettage, endometrial jet washing, intrauterine nylon brushes or scrapers and the use of the hysteroscope. Unfortunately, it has not been possible to apply any of these techniques on a large scale.

Perhaps the most practical step towards earlier diagnosis is to educate the public to seek medical advice should they have any post-menopausal bleeding or any irregular bleeding around the time of the menopause and to provide efficient outpatient and hospital services where these complaints can be investigated.

Pathology

The tumour is nearly always an adeno-carcinoma which spreads around the endometrium, projects into the cavity and eventually invades the myometrium. Sometimes the malignant change is confined to one small area of the endometrium and this makes thorough and complete curettage essential for diagnosis. Most tumours are well-differentiated and the papillary type is common. The more highly differentiated the tumour, the better the prognosis. Adeno-acanthoma is a tumour with areas of squamous metaplasia. Its prognosis does not differ from that of papillary adeno-carcinoma and its treatment is the same. Adeno-squamous carcinomas are tumours which contain almost equal amounts of squamous and glandular components. They are comparatively rare but are of importance as their prognosis is said to be poor. Endometrial adeno-carcinoma remains confined to the uterus until a comparatively late stage. While it is still localised to the endometrium it usually manifests itself by the notable symptom of post-menopausal bleeding and this makes effective treatment possible before it has spread too far.

When the tumour spreads through the myometrium it may also involve the tube, ovary and the pelvic peritoneum.

A useful staging of endometrial carcinoma is as follows:

Stage I: Carcinoma confined to the corpus uteri.
1. Not invading the myometrium.
2. Invading the myometrium to one third of its thickness.
3. Invading the myometrium to two thirds of its thickness.
4. Penetrating the uterine serosa.

Stage II: Carcinoma involving the corpus and the cervix.

Stage III: Carcinoma extending outside the uterus but not outside the true pelvis.

Stage IV: Carcinoma extending outside the true pelvis or involving bladder or rectum.

Clinical features

The symptom of endometrial cancer is abnormal bleeding and because of the age of the patients this is usually post-menopausal. Occasionally the first symptom in an elderly woman may be a watery discharge or a purulent discharge associated with a pyometra. In pre-menopausal women the bleeding is usually intermenstrual, but any pattern of bleeding may be associated with carcinoma. On examination many patients are noted to be obese. Many have atrophic vaginitis and uterine enlargement is seldom found. Rarely, the disease may present with vaginal metastases on first examination. Metastases in lungs or bones are late features.

Diagnosis

Diagnosis must always be made by histological examination of uterine curettings, preferably by an experienced gynaecological pathologist, for difficulties in interpretation are fairly frequent. Dilatation and curettage for post-menopausal bleeding should always be done with great care, preferably by an experienced gynaecologist or under his direct supervision, because it is easy to perforate the soft thin uterine wall. The whole uterine cavity must be carefully explored. If the tumour is invading the myometrium the characteristic rough scrape of the curette on the muscle will be absent and the instrument will feel as if it is passing over soft material like cheese. Fractional curettage, where the endocervix is curetted first, is found useful by some, but not all are agreed that it is useful in deciding the precise site of the lesion.

Treatment

The basic treatment is surgical. Total hysterectomy and bilateral salpingo-oophorectomy will give a five-year survival rate of 60 per cent, but there will be a number of recurrences in the vault of the vagina probably caused by spill of cancer cells during the operation. Various methods have been devised to improve results by preventing these local metastases and the principal one is the use of radiotherapy as an adjuvant to surgery. The main argument about radiotherapy is whether it should be given before or after operation. Pre-operative intra-cavitary and vault radium is the most fashionable form of treatment as it is thought to inactivate the cancer before proceeding to surgery. Unfortunately it also prevents the pathologist from making detailed assessment of the tissues he receives in the laboratory. If, for example, no cancer is found, is that because of the radiotherapy or because of the preliminary curettage?

Surgeons who operate one week after the application of radium claim there is no technical difficulty but as a general principle it is probably best to avoid cutting and stitching irradiated tissues. My own preference is to make the primary treatment surgical, removing the uterus, tubes, ovaries and as much of the vault of the vagina as possible (for access is often difficult in obese patients). The para-aortic lymph nodes are palpated carefully to detect any involvement and the abdomen is closed. Once the abdominal wound has healed post-operative radiation can be given in the light of a full report by the pathologist.

The most common method is the insertion of vaginal radium which can be done several weeks after operation. Alternatively, or additionally, the patient can have a course of 20 treatments of external deep X-ray therapy to the pelvis in the same manner as for carcinoma of the cervix.

Attempts have been made to improve results in endometrial carcinoma by performing the Wertheim operation as a primary treatment but although expert surgeons can produce good results from this, the incidence of lymph node involvement is too low to justify the use of this radical procedure in elderly and sometimes unfit patients. A few patients who are unfit for surgery may be treated by radiotherapy alone, by packing the uterine cavity with Heyman's capsules, following this by external super-voltage radiation to the whole pelvis. Results from this treatment in selected cases are by no means unreasonable.

Progestogen treatment has been used for nearly 20 years and was introduced in the hope of ameliorating extensive disease, such as metastases in the lungs. The way in which progestational agents bring about an objective remission in endometrial cancer (which they undoubtedly can do) is not well understood; they may act locally on individual tumour cells or it may depress the production of some natural tumour-stimulating substance.

Any potent progestational agent seems to be as effective as another in producing a remission in secondary endometrial carcinoma.

Agents given orally, intramuscularly or into the cavity of the uterus have all produced equally good effects.

It has also been suggested that progestational agents may be of value in the prophylaxis of endometrial cancer, but this is very difficult to prove.

CARCINOMA OF THE OVARY

Carcinoma of the ovary is the commonest gynaecological cancer. It causes more than 3000 deaths in England and Wales each year, which is about the same number as the deaths from cancer of the cervix and cancer of the endometrium combined.

Mortality from ovarian cancer seems to be increasing at a rate of about 15 per cent per decade.

Nearly 2 per cent of all women may be expected ultimately to die of cancer of the ovary. Most deaths occur in women in their fifties and sixties and the incidence appears to be higher in single than in married women.

The overall five-year survival rate from cancer of the ovary is only about 30 per cent in most areas, largely because of delay in making the diagnosis.

No carcinogenic agent can be identified and it is perhaps more constructive to think of ovarian cancer not as a single entity but as a group of diseases which may have different aetiologies.

Pathology
There is no organ which produces so many and varied tumours as the ovary. The classification and polysyllabic nomenclature of these tumours is quite bewildering to the clinician and detailed pathological discussions tend to generate more heat than light. The pathology of ovarian tumours is further confused by cystic changes which may develop as a result of the physiological activity of the ovary.

Ovarian cancers may be cystic or solid. They are bilateral in 25 per cent of cases. Some of the more important varieties are:

1. *Primary cystic carcinoma of the ovary.* This may arise *de novo* or develop from a previously benign cyst. It may be serous or mucinous in type. Serous cystadenocarcinoma is more common

than the mucinous variety and is often of papillary type. It tends to implant early on the peritoneum and to produce ascites. Mucinous cystadenocarcinoma grossly resemble benign mucinous cysts but usually have more solid areas: histology shows a typical adenocarcinoma in which mucinous elements are generally retained.

2. *Primary solid carcinoma of the ovary.* This is usually an adenocarcinoma with various degrees of differentiation. The histology may sometimes resemble endometrial carcinoma.

Other solid carcinomas have no adenomatus pattern. Solid ovarian cancers seldom attain great size but they may fill the pelvis. The opened tumour may show to the naked eye a greyish appearance and its consistency is variable.

3. *Secondary carcinoma of the ovary.* The ovary is a common site of metastasis, mainly from the breast and the gastro-intestinal tract.

One specific type of secondary carcinoma is the Krukenberg tumour which is almost always associated with gastro-intestinal malignancy. The tumours are almost always bilateral and are solid. Histology shows striking stromal proliferation and small nests or acini of epithelial cells many of which show the characteristic 'signet ring' form caused by mucoid degeneration pushing the flattened nucleus against one side of the cell.

4. *Granulosa cell tumour.* This is the commonest of the sex cord ovarian tumours and accounts for 9 per cent of primary ovarian carcinomas. It is usually a tumour of reproductive years but may cause precocious puberty. The tumour is unilateral in 95 per cent of cases and is sometimes very small. Histologically the tumours are diagnosed by the presence of cords or rosettes of granulosa cells.

5. *Dysgerminoma.* This is a germ cell tumour and is structurally identical with the seminoma in the male. It usually has no endocrine function. It occurs most commonly in young women with an average age of 18 (hence the old name 'carcinoma puellarum'). Occasionally, dysgerminomas are found in patients with gonadal dysgenesis. Dysgerminomas are usually unilateral, they are solid, greyish in colour and usually show no sign of extension. Histology shows large round cells with dark staining nuclei and abundant cytoplasm: these cells are arranged in clumps divided by fibrous septa. There is considerable doubt about the degree of malignancy of the dysgerminoma but there is no doubt that it is malignant.

Staging

The stage of extension which ovarian cancers reach is much more important for prognosis than the histological grade or type of tumour. The staging of ovarian cancer proposed by the International Federation of Obstetrics and Gynaecology (FIGO) is as follows:

Stage I:	Growth limited to the ovaries.
Ia	Growth limited to one ovary: no ascites.
	(i) Capsule not ruptured (ii) Capsule ruptured.
Ib	Growth limited to both ovaries; no ascites.
	(i) Capsule not ruptured (ii) Capsule ruptured.
Ic	Growth limited to one or both ovaries: ascites present with malignant cells in the fluid.
	(i) Capsule not ruptured (ii) Capsule ruptured.
Stage II:	Growth involving one or both ovaries with pelvic extension.
IIa	Extension and metastasis to uterus and tubes only.
IIb	Extension to other pelvic tissues.
Stage III:	Growth involving one or both ovaries with widespread intraperitoneal metastases.
Stage IV:	Growth involving one or both ovaries with distant metastases.

The staging of ovarian tumours throws into sharp relief the urgent need for early diagnosis. Usually, more than two thirds of the patients present when the growth has already reached Stages III or IV and their survival rate for five years is approximately 10 per cent.

Clinical features
Clinical features are usually late in making their appearance. It is possible, however, for the gynaecologist always to bear in mind the possibility of ovarian cancer in every patient whom he examines and in this way he may hope to pick up early tumours. Many patients come for a cervical smear, for contraceptive advice or for a diagnostic curettage and if all these patients have a careful pelvic examination, there is a hope that some early tumours may be revealed. Any adnexal mass should be viewed as a possible cancer until proved benign and the detection of a pelvic mass or palpable ovary in a post-menopausal woman should suggest strongly the possibility of ovarian cancer.

Laparoscopy should be performed if the findings are doubtful: if the findings on pelvic examination are positive, laparotomy should be done, following the old adage –

'Lump = cut   :   No lump = no cut'.

It is only when the abdomen is open that the diagnosis of the nature of an ovarian tumour can be made and in some cases even later for detailed histological examination may take some time.

The *symptoms* most commonly related by sufferers from ovarian carcinoma are abdominal pain, abdominal swelling and abnormal vaginal bleeding.

The history is often of an indefinite nature and the patient's first visit to hospital may be not to a gynaecologist but to a general physician or surgeon. Medical students should be taught that ovarian carcinoma is one of the commonest causes of abdominal swelling in middle-aged women and that the tumour is often the underlying cause of ascites.

The physical *signs* are those of a pelvic tumour and there may be little change to signify the transformation from a benign to a malignant cyst. Ovarian cancers seldom attain the enormous size of the mucinous cysts which fill the whole abdomen and have attracted much attention from Ephraim McDowell onwards. Such huge tumours are usually benign. However, carcinomas of the ovary may be of substantial size – sometimes that of a melon and their malignant nature may be suspected by fixity, the presence of ascites and the characteristic nodular deposits in the Pouch of Douglas. The gynaecologist must always remember that the ovarian cancer could be a secondary one.

Pre-operative investigations are unlikely to lead to any more precise diagnosis than clinical examination but a full blood count, liver function tests, urea and electrolytes, a chest X-ray and an intravenous pyelogram will be useful, while in some cases where bowel disease is suspected, barium enema and sigmoidoscopy will be necessary.

Sonar will confirm the outline of any ovarian tumour but signs of malignant change will only be present when they are macroscopically obvious; solid areas may be seen projecting into a cystic tumour, there may be a bizarre echo pattern and associated ascites will be detected. Hepatic metastases may be demonstrated by grey-scale technique and it may be possible to monitor the effect of treatment on their size by ultrasonic means.

Treatment

The primary treatment of ovarian cancer is surgical. Laparotomy should be done in practically every case for only then can the true situation be assessed and many patients can have their symptoms relieved at least temporarily. Radiotherapy or chemotherapy should not be given blindly no matter how certain the diagnosis may seem clinically or on tests such as the cytology of ascitic fluid. Laparotomy will usually establish the precise diagnosis, will allow staging of the growth and will provide initial treatment by enabling the surgeon to remove as much of the tumour as possible. In Stages I and II, total hysterectomy, bilateral salpingo-oophorectomy and omentectomy should be performed and a careful inspection of the pelvic peritoneum and palpation of the liver should be done to exclude secondaries. Removal of the omentum is a valuable procedure for microscopic secondaries may be found in it. In the later stages of ovarian carcinoma there are often large omental plaques of tumour and their removal aids further treatment. The general principle in operating on Stages III and IV should be to remove as much tumour tissue as can be done with safety to the patient. Reduction in the bulk of the tumour helps to control ascites and probably improves the response to subsequent radiotherapy or chemotherapy.

Ovarian carcinoma is an extremely unpredictable disease and occasionally some patients (especially the elderly) seem to get completely better after simple surgery despite unfavourable findings at laparotomy. However, the general prognosis is poor and it is usually the practice to supplement surgery with abdominal radiotherapy or systemic chemotherapy.

Total abdominal radiation involves giving about 2500 rads by external megavoltage therapy in about 20 divided doses. Treatment can be started as soon as the abdomen is healed.

The methods of giving systemic chemotherapy are almost as many as the drugs themselves. Chemotherapy is the only way of managing advanced disease after surgery and radiotherapy or of treating widespread recurrence.

Chlorambucil, cyclophosphamide, melphalan and triethylenethiophosphoramide are the most commonly used alkylating agents and seem to be equally effective.

Among non-alkylating agents 5-Fluorouracil has been the most extensively used, but many patients have also been treated with methotrexate and vinblastine and vincristine. Adriamycin is now being employed increasingly and seems to have some therapeutic effect.

Combination chemotherapy is now popular and the various drug regimes require skilled supervision by those expert in their use. Immunotherapy is also being tried but is at the experimental stage.

The great problem with all forms of treatment of ovarian carcinoma is to make an objective assessment of their efficacy. Attempts at some form of controlled trial are at present being made but the unpredictability and varied nature of the tumours involved must always be remembered.

A special problem arises when ovarian carcinoma is diagnosed in a young nulliparous woman. There is a great temptation to be conservative and to preserve her ability to have children. This is probably a mistake for it is impossible to be sure that the other ovary does not harbour a microscopic tumour.

Patients with advanced and recurrent ovarian carcinoma are likely to suffer distress from abdominal distension from ascitic fluid or gas. Ascites can be dealt with by repeated paracentesis but gaseous distension may eventually proceeed to intestinal obstruction. Prolonged gastric suction and intravenous drip are often surprisingly successful in controlling the bowel symptoms and an unnecessary laparotomy should be avoided whenever possible. To the patient with advanced ovarian cancer the quality of the nursing care she receives is more important than any operation or chemotherapeutic drug.

Junior medical staff and nurses should be instructed carefully in the management of these patients whom they cannot cure but can do so much to relieve.

CHORIOCARCINOMA

This is a highly malignant tumour which, in about half the cases follows hydatidiform mole. About a quarter of the cases are preceded by normal pregnancy and another quarter by abortion or ectopic pregnancy. Choriocarcinoma is a very vascular tumour containing cells resembling those of chorionic trophoblast. Non-malignant theca-lutein cysts may be present in the ovaries. Chorio-carcinoma can metastasise widely especially to the lungs and vagina. 75 per cent of hydatidiform moles develop some invasive properties but only 3 per cent of these fail to regress within 6 months. If these malignant cases are treated by chemotherapy within the following 6 months there is virtually 100 per cent cure.

After delivery or removal of a hydatidiform mole, quantitative tests for chorionic gonadotrophin (HCG) in serum or urine are performed at the following times:

1. Three weeks post evacuation.
2. Every two weeks until HCG levels are normal.
3. Every month until one year post-evacuation.
4. Every three months until two years post-evacuation.
5. Three weeks after any subsequent pregnancy.

If the HCG test becomes positive again or if there is abnormal vaginal bleeding choriocarcinoma should be suspected and may be revealed on curettage. The lungs should be X-rayed for metastases. Less than one per cent of patients who have had normal HCG levels in the first year have a rise in level in the second year and none have been recorded in the third year. It seems reasonable to stop follow-up at 2 years.

Women with high HCG levels who are taking the contraceptive pill have a higher incidence of trophoblastic disease, therefore oral contraception should not be used until one month after HCG levels are normal. If the HCG levels are normal for six months, the patient can be advised that it is safe to conceive. Follow-up of hydatidiform mole should be precise and is best organised by special centres. Choriocarcinoma and its metastases respond to treatment with folic acid antagonists (e.g. Methotrexate 0·5 mg/kg daily for five days). Courses of this often combined with other chemotherapeutic drugs are repeated unless there are severe toxic symptoms or agranulocytosis. Modern specialised chemotherapy has converted what was once a greatly feared malignant tumour into a curable disease. Cases of choriocarcinoma should be referred to special centres for the best results.

16

Prolapse and urinary incontinence

Prolapse of the uterus and vaginal walls is one of the commonest conditions treated by the gynaecologist. Utero-vaginal prolapse is often accompanied by urinary symptoms. Prolapse does not endanger life but interferes greatly with liberty and the pursuit of happiness because it restricts mobility, demoralises the patient with constant discomfort and, particularly if urinary symptoms are present, may render her unable to work efficiently or enjoy a reasonable social life.

The relief of the symptoms of prolapse is one of the great triumphs of gynaecology. The very fact that this relief is so often achieved by simple vaginal operations employing basic surgical principles and a modicum of skill should not detract from recognition of its importance. Much attention is paid in the medical literature to arguments about operative technique and much is also written about problem cases of urinary incontinence but the fact is that most patients are successfully treated by methods which have stood the test of time and should be respected for their efficiency.

Aetiology of prolapse

The uterus is maintained in its normal position by anatomical supports inserted around the level of the cervix, chiefly the transverse cervical and uterosacral ligaments. The pubo-cervical fascia helps to support the bladder and at a lower level the muscles of the pelvic floor give further support to the internal organs. It is well known that, in patients with complete perineal tears where the pelvic floor muscles are forced to be very active to produce some degree of rectal continence, prolapse is particularly unknown.

The main factors causing prolapse are:

1. *Congenital weakness of uterine supports.*This explains the occasional occurrence of prolapse in the nulliparous patient and is an important factor in other cases.

2. *Birth trauma*. The patient may give no overt history of

traumatic deliveries but there is no doubt that childbirth is the main cause. Stretching the uterine supports combined with damage to the cervix and perineum are the initial lesions which are later aggravated by menopausal atrophy.

3. *Menopausal changes.* The hormone deficiencies of the post-menopausal years cause atrophic changes in the genital tract and prolapse then becomes manifest and gives rise to symptoms.

4. *Raised intra-abdominal pressure.* The main causes of this are obesity and chronic bronchitis (in other words, over-indulgence in food and tobacco). Raised intra-abdominal pressure is a very important contributory factor.

Symptoms of prolapse

The symptoms of prolapse do not always correlate with the physical signs. For example, some women with gross prolapse have no symptoms at all, while others with minimal anatomical defects seem to suffer acute discomfort. The theory has been advanced that extensive cases of prolapse may be associated with stretching and disruption of nerve fibres with resultant insensitivity but this is probably not the whole explanation. Psychosomatic causes, as with all diseases, influence the timing and manner of the patient's complaint.

The characteristic of all symptoms of prolapse is that they are worse when the woman is up and about and get better when she lies down. If this feature is not present it is unlikely that prolapse is the cause of the symptoms. Symptoms of prolapse can be classified as non-urinary and urinary.

Non-urinary symptoms

The most common is a feeling of discomfort in the vagina, traditionally described as 'something coming down'. There may be associated backache and lower abdominal discomfort. In extensive cases a lump may protrude outside the introitus and this may give rise to discharge, ulceration and bleeding. Carcinoma of the cervix is strangely rare in cases of prolapse. A large rectocele may cause difficulty in defaecation and bowel emptying may need to be completed by digital pressure on the rectocele. Gross prolapses sometimes become incarcerated and are then oedematous and painful: they can usually be reduced by skilful manual replacement, sometimes after some hours of postural treatment, with the lower end of the bed raised.

Urinary symptoms

The main ones are frequency, urgency and stress incontinence.

Frequency cannot be assumed to be due to prolapse (e.g. cysto-cele) unless urinary tract pathology is excluded. Infection is the commonest cause of increased frequency.

Urgency may be a feature in some cases of cystocele and urethro-cele. It is unlikely to be cured by a vaginal repair operation unless visible laxity is present. Like frequency, urgency may be caused by cystitis. It may also be a manifestation of 'detrusor instability'.

Stress incontinence is defined as the escape of a little urine through the intact urethra when the intra-abdominal pressure is raised as by coughing or laughing. Stress incontinence is the commonest urinary symptom in post-menopausal women. The gynaecologist must remember, when assessing symptoms, that leakage of a little urine may occur occasionally in women of all ages: his duty is to find out if his patient's symptom is sufficiently troublesome to warrant treatment. Stress incontinence is caused by weakness or incompetence of the bladder neck (at the junction of bladder and urethra) which should normally be closed, compe-tent and able to resist the strain of increased intra-abdominal pressure. If the bladder neck is incompetent, an increase in intra-abdominal pressure reverses the normal closure gradient between bladder and urethra so that incontinence occurs.

The symptom or sign of stress incontinence does not confirm a sphincter weakness as the cause but is very suggestive of it. Lack of support to the urethra is an important cause of sphincter weak-ness and there may be a demonstrable widening of the normal angle between the urethra and the base of the bladder.

Retention of urine may occur in cases where the urethra is well supported but there is a large cystocele hanging down below it, the urethra then being rather like the spout on a teapot. Sometimes the patient may have to push the cystocele up in order to void urine. Sometimes there is overflow incontinence with a substantial amount of residual urine. This is the state of affairs known to the urologists as 'outflow obstruction'. The absence of residual urine does not exclude outflow obstruction for a hypertrophical detrusor muscle may produce a sufficiently high voiding pressure to empty the bladder.

Clinical signs of prolapse and urinary incontinence
Having taken the history and formed a general idea of the patient's complaints and the disability they are causing the gynaecologist proceeds to the usual clinical examination. This may be conducted with the patient in the dorsal or lateral position. (The lateral

position as Sims showed long ago is the ideal one for visualising prolapse of the anterior wall).

In both these positions the patient is recumbent and as the symptoms of prolapse are always worse when the woman stands up, the limitations of the usual clinical examination should be remembered, particularly when it comes to the assessment of urinary symptoms.

Examination begins with inspection and a large prolapse and extensive deficiency of the perineum may be immediately visible. The patient is then asked to cough: this may bring down a cystocele, rectocele or enterocele and may demonstrate stress incontinence. Demonstrable stress incontinence merely confirms the history of urinary leakage given by the patient without indicating its cause and failure to produce urinary leakage at the time of examination does not mean that her complaint is not a genuine one. If digital pressure to elevate the tissues at the sides of the urethra (without obstructing the urethra itself) succeeds in controlling the incontinence this augurs well for the success of a repair operation. Retraction of the perineum with the patient in the lateral position will give a good view of the anterior vaginal wall and cervix from which a smear should be taken. The presence of atrophic vaginitis or of scarring from previous operations should be noted. While prolapse of the vaginal walls (urethrocele and cystocele anteriorly and rectocele and enterocele posteriorly) may occur without much uterine descent, prolapse of the uterus itself seldom occurs on its own. It is customary to classify uterine prolapse in three stages:

Stage I: The cervix comes down to the introitus
Stage II: The cervix is outside the introitus
Stage III: The whole uterus is outside the introitus

In Stage II there is often hypertrophic elongation of the supra-vaginal cervix which can be felt between the examiner's finger and thumb as a firm continuous structure (rather like the neck of a chicken) going up into the abdomen. In Stage III the whole uterus is outside, lying in a bag of everted vagina and the examiner's finger and thumb can meet above the fundus.

Assessment of fitness for operation
Having made the diagnosis of the local gynaecological condition an evaluation of the patient's general fitness should be made, with special reference to her cardiac and respiratory function. Many patients with prolapse are elderly, may are obese, many are hyper-

tensive but these disabilities may not debar them from getting great benefit from operation, although they undoubtedly increase its risks.

The gynaecologist must first decide whether the patient's symptoms are caused by uterovaginal prolapse and secondly whether they are severe enough to justify operation. If the answer to these questions is 'yes' the help of physician and anaesthetist may be necessary in deciding the question of fitness for operation.

With modern anaesthesia there are few patients who are unfit for at least some form of surgery. The actual operation to be performed should be chosen with care and performed skilfully and expeditiously with the minimum amount of bleeding and disruption of the tissues.

Non-operative treatment

This may be tried in the young fit woman still in the childbearing years and may be the only resort for some elderly women with severe medical disabilities.

The young woman. Young women with prolapse may have to wear a pessary in the early months of pregnancy but after the uterus enlarges to become an abdominal organ the pessary can be removed. After delivery, intensive physiotherapy should be employed. The patient actually treats herself by developing voluntary control of the pelvic floor muscles. This is best demonstrated to her by the gynaecologist retracting the perineum with two fingers and then showing the patient how to pull up her pelvic floor against the examining fingers, telling her to contract her muscles as if she were trying to prevent her bowels from moving. Voluntary elevation of the perineum also produces elevation of the anterior vaginal wall and may help urethral closure: assiduous practice may cure or greatly relieve stress incontinence.

If no benefit is obtained after a reasonable trial of physiotherapy over a number of months there should be no hesitation in proceeding to operate despite the patient's youth rather than leaving her in misery till the menopause or even after.

The elderly and unfit. The elderly and unfit may be relieved by oestrogen therapy and by insertion of pessaries. People with minimal degrees of prolapse and some with troublesome urinary symptoms sometimes get remarkable relief from oestrogens, given either locally or systemically. Oestrogen treatment is also useful as a pre-operative measure particularly if atrophic vaginitis is present.

Those who are unfit for operation or refuse it can be kept comfortable with a flexible plastic ring pessary of suitable size. Modern inert plastics do not cause so much irritation and discharge as the older types, but should be changed every 3 months and the vagina inspected carefully for any ulceration.

Special investigations and treatment of urinary incontinence

Sometimes patients with troublesome incontinence have very little evidence of prolapse; a few patients may already have had a vaginal repair operation with an apparently good anatomical result. These patients need investigations to find out the cause of the incontinence and to select the correct method of treatment. Such investigations demand the special skills of the urologist and in some centres combined 'urodynamic clinic' have been established to deal with the problem of incontinence.

Basic urological investigations
These are necessary before any urodynamic studies are done.
Culture of the urine. Culture of the urine may show evidence of infection; recurrent bacteruria may be a cause of recurrent dysuria frequency and urgency, and an attempt should be made to sterilise the urine.
Intravenous pyelography. This is essential to exclude stone, tuberculosis and congenital anomalies.
Cystoscopy and urethroscopy. These arts require long and careful training. Cystoscopy will diagnose or exclude conditions such as stone, bladder tumours, carcinoma-*in-situ* or interstitial cystitis while urethroscopy will note the presence or absence of diverticula.

Urodynamic investigations
Urodynamic investigations have proved an aid to diagnosis in difficult cases.
Cystometry. Cystometry is the fundamental method of assessing detrusor function and detecting detrusor instability. This investigation is best performed on a tilting table in an X-ray department. The total bladder pressure and rectal pressure are measured using a two channel recording system. The intrinsic detrusor pressure is the difference between the total bladder pressure and the rectal pressure. This measurement gives the best indication of detrusor activity.

If the cystometrogram is abnormal a search should be made for a neuropathy – e.g. disseminsated sclerosis or cord compression by enlarged inter-laminar joints in lumbar spondylosis.

Detrusor instability is a major cause of frequency nocturia and urge incontinence: in most cases there is no overt neurological abnormality but the existence of the symptoms suggests some upset in neural control. Many cases have a psychosomatic element.

Voiding flow studies. Voiding flow studies may demonstrate bladder outlet obstruction, but this is a relatively uncommon diagnosis in women, unlike men who often suffer from prostatic obstruction. In those women who have true urethral obstruction, dilatation or urethrotomy may be beneficial.

Treatment. Most patients with urinary problems get at least some benefit from conservative procedures and these should be tried first before resorting to surgery unless an operation is indicated for prolapse in a case where the urinary symptoms are only a part of the general clinical picture.

General rules of health. Rules of health such as weight reduction and avoidance of smoking should be enforced first. This is easier said than done, particularly in this self indulgent and anti-authoritarian age.

Oestrogen therapy. This will reverse atrophic changes in the vagina and urethra and this simple treatment is often surprisingly successful in curing urinary symptoms.

Anticholinergic drugs. Anticholinergic drugs such as probanthine hydrochloride and imipramine and anti-spasmodics such as flavoxate hydrochloride may be useful. The action of these drugs may be aided by a tranquiliser such as diazepam.

Bladder drill. If enforced strictly this may bring about a cure of detrusor instability and if the patient is unable to produce an improvement by voluntary effort prolonged bladder distension under epidural block may be useful.

Mechanical and electrical devices. Various such devices have been used to aid bladder control but have not yet had wide acceptance.

Surgery. Surgery is discussed in association with the surgery of prolapse, for most patients for whom operation is indicated – i.e. those with vesico-urethral displacement and deficient support – benefit from a vaginal repair. Occasionally there are patients (particularly those who have had previous operations) for whom it seems that a vaginal repair would be inappropriate. They may benefit from one of the special operations devised for urinary incontinence. The Aldridge sling operation uses an abdomino-vaginal approach and the sling is made from strips of fascia from the external oblique aponeurosia. It is very difficult to achieve a good result and perfect tension in the sling. These comments also apply to the gauze-hammock operation devised by Chassar Moir. The Marshall-Marchetti-Krantz operation (vesico-urethropexy) involves an abdominal approach with stitching of the tissues at the sides of the urethra to the back of the symphysis pubis – this may sometimes be effective, but there is a risk of osteitis pubis. Colposuspension is a similar retropubic procedure, where the lateral vaginal fornices are suspended to the ileopectineal line. Mulvany's operation (urethro-vesicolysis) involves a different principle from the previous two which fix the bladder and urethra – namely freeing the bladder and urethra from surrounding adhesions.

The average gynaecological surgeon who is competent in vaginal repair work has few opportunities to acquire skill in these special techniques and there is much to be said for referring problem cases to specialist centres.

Operations for utero-vaginal prolapse

The operation best suited for a particular patient must be chosen after careful consideration of the anatomical nature of the displacement and of the symptoms it causes.

Good results depend greatly on the selection of cases and on surgical skill.

Vaginal operations devised from knowledge of the supporting functions of the transverse cervical and uterosacral ligaments and aimed at the restoration of normal anatomy are likely to be successful. From the practical point of view there are three main types of operation:

1. Anterior colporrhaphy and/or colpoperineorrhaphy are indicated for simple vaginal prolapse with minimal descent of the vault in young women who are likely to have further children or in some older patients with similar defects where simplicity and speed are desired.
2. The Manchester or Donald-Fothergill operation is indicated for uterovaginal prolapse where there is descent of the cervix and vault as well as cystocele and/or rectocele. In this operation, in addition to anterior colporrhaphy and/or colpoperineorrhaphy, the cervix is amputated and the lax cardinal ligaments shortened. A posterior repair is not necessary in every case: if the perineum is reasonably normal and no rectocele or enterocele is present a colpoperineorrhaphy may succeed only in causing dyspareunia. Efficient support of the vaginal vault is the main feature of the Manchester operation.
3. Vaginal hysterectomy and pelvic floor repair is an alternative to the Manchester operation and may be indicated in patients

who desire a sterilising operation or who suffer from uterine pathology such as dysfunctional bleeding, small fibroids or dysplasia of the cervix. Vaginal hysterectomy is the operation of choice in the elderly patient with complete procidentia and a hernia of the pouch of Douglas. It must be emphasised that removal of the uterus in itself does nothing to cure prolapse. The treatment of genital prolapse requires a repair of the weakened tissues of the pelvic floor and hysterectomy may be incidental to this procedure.

The end results of both the Manchester operation and vaginal hysterectomy, in terms of curing prolapse and leaving a functional vagina, can be equally good.

Operations for vesico-vaginal fistula

Vesico-vaginal fistula produces complete urinary incontinence and the life of a patient with this disability is miserable indeed. Fistulas caused by obstetric trauma are seldom seen in countries where maternity services are well developed. Urinary fistulas can generally be diagnosed by colouring the urine with a dye such as Methylene Blue. Small fistulas may close spontaneously with bladder drainage and several months may be allowed to pass in some cases before attempting surgery. Operations for fistulae are specialised procedures but certain basic principles are involved in all of them. These include freedom from local sepsis, adequate exposure, excision of fibrous tissue from the edges, approximation of the edges without tension, the use of suitable suture material and efficient post-operative bladder drainage.

Complications of repair operations

1. *Haemorrhage* during operation may be minimised by gentle handling of the tissues and avoidance of unnecessary dissection and opening of tissue planes. If fresh bleeding occurs in the first 24 hours after operation the patient should be taken back to theatre immediately so that the bleeding point can be identified and haemostasis secured. At a later stage a haematoma may form. This can generally be treated conservatively but it may be very debilitating for the patient.

2. *Urinary retention* is the commonest post-operative complication. Careful recording of liquid intake and output is essential. If the bladder is full, overflow incontinence may occur and this may be deceptive. Medical and nursing staff should be taught to palpate the abdomen to detect the full bladder. The use of indwelling catheters should be avoided

where possible as they cause a high rate of urinary infection.

3. *Pelvic infection* may occur, often due to infection in a haematoma. Antibiotic treatment usually deals with this satisfactorily and the infected haematoma tends to drain spontaneously.

4. *Thrombosis and embolism* may result in death. This fact must always be remembered when advising surgery for a condition which may cause much discomfort but does not threaten life. The prophylactic use of anticoagulants is discussed elsewhere.

5. *Dyspareunia* can occur because of excessive narrowing of the vagina. The statement is sometimes made that it is justifiable to narrow the vagina in elderly women or widows. This view sets a poor standard for the art of vaginal surgery. The aim should be to restore normal anatomy as nearly as possible. If dyspareunia occurs after operation it can usually be treated by a combination of oestrogen creams and vaginal dilators without resort to further surgery.

6. *Cervical stenosis* may occur after amputation. It can cause haematometra or, more important, difficulties in labour. At the worst a tear of the stenosed cervix can result in uterine rupture and death. For this reason, all women who have had repair operations involving cervical amputation and who subsequently become pregnant should be delivered by caesarean section.

17

Post-operative complications

Post-operative complications may be minimised by careful selection and pre-operative assessment of the patient, by careful technique in theatre, by the use of specialised recovery wards where the patient receives intensive observation during the first few hours of operation (under clear instructions given by the surgeon and the anaesthetist) and by careful attention to clinical detail and routine in the wards thereafter. Any operation, however, carries with it the risk of complications. These may be *local* involving the operation site itself, or *general* affecting any of the other systems of the body; they may be *immediate*, within the first 24 hours of operation, *early* within the first two or three weeks after operation, or *late* often weeks or months after the patient has left hospital.

LOCAL COMPLICATIONS

Gynaecological operations involve wounds in the abdomen or vagina or both. Hysterectomy is an operation performed in a contaminated field. Abdominal hysterectomy involves wounds in both abdomen and vagina, but vaginal hysterectomy tends to have the higher incidence of febrile morbidity after operation, probably because of the large numbers of endogenous potentially pathogenic organisms in the vagina.

Haematoma

A haematoma is likely to form if haemostasis in every layer of the wound is not complete. A deep haematoma may give rise to severe pain and shock and any haematoma other than the smallest is likely to be associated with a rise in pulse rate and temperature. The wound is tense and tender and there may be marked superficial bruising. Sub-cutaneous haematomas in the abdominal wall may be allowed to evacuate spontaneously, particularly if a low transverse incision has been employed for the operation, but deep haematomas may require surgical evacuation.

Wound infection

The patient with an infected wound is still in pain and has a fever. There is brawny induration of the wound and an abscess may point in it. If pus forms it should be drained. Infection in a haematoma is probably the most important single cause of suppuration in both abdominal and vaginal wounds.

Specific vaginal wound complications

The patient who has had a vaginal hysterectomy or Manchester repair operation has incisions in the vagina and may have a perineal wound also if a posterior repair has been performed. A certain amount of discharge which is initially blood-stained and later purulent is to be expected after all these operations and the patient should be reassured that it is a normal feature. All patients who have had vaginal hysterectomies or repairs should have a gentle vaginal examination made before discharge from hospital to confirm that no foreign body is present and to separate any light adhesions that may have formed between the suture lines. Adhesions may be a cause of late complications from vaginal operations particularly if scar tissue becomes organised. Another late complication of great importance to the patient may be vaginal stenosis. Colpoperineorrhaphy is the main cause of stenosis after vaginal repair operations. In some cases it may be possible to cure the patient's symptoms without performing a posterior repair and, in any case, it is advisable to avoid over enthusiastic stitching of the perineum, but in patients with recurrent prolapse whose symptoms are very troublesome, it may be impossible to preserve the function of the vagina and at the same time to give the patient an efficient surgical cure. Such patients must be warned of the possibility of vaginal stenosis and they may be prepared to face this in the interest of relief of their complaint particularly if it is one of urinary incontinence.

Rupture of the abdominal wound

This may be caused by factors existing before the operation such as extensive carcinoma, by factors connected with faulty operative technique, or by factors occurring after the operation, such as coughing, flatulent distension of the abdomen and haematoma formation. In some cases, the rupture may be complete and traumatic with loops of bowel appearing through the wound. This not unnaturally causes mortal fear. Often wound rupture is more insidious and a discharge of blood-stained serous fluid from the wound may indicate that the peritoneal suture line is open. It is important that every attempt should be made at operation to produce a watertight closure of the peritoneum and, if necessary, the peritoneum should be mobilised to produce close apposition of the edges without tension. If signs of wound dehiscence are apparent, resuture should be performed preferably using non-absorbable materials through all layers except the peritoneum.

Foreign bodies in the abdomen or vagina
The most common of these is a swab and this may give rise to serious medical and legal complications. It is essential that swabs containing a radio-opaque thread should be used throughout. It is better to work with large swabs and to use as few as possible. This makes efficient swab counting easier. Swabs are particularly liable to be left behind in the course of emergency and perhaps life-saving operations when there may be some haste and confusion. The presence of swabs in the vagina can be excluded by careful examination at the end of the operation and again before dismissal and if there is suspicion of a swab being left in the abdomen at any time during the post-operative period, the patient should have an X-ray. It is unusual for instruments to be left inside the abdomen but it is more easy to mislay small instruments than large ones; long handled instruments are best for pelvic surgery. Drains or pieces of them may sometimes be retained in the abdomen but this is unlikely if they are transfixed with sutures to the skin and are removed completely in 48 hours.

Incisional hernia
This is a late complication. It is uncommon when the low transverse incision is used for abdominal operations. It is more commonly associated with mid-line and para-median incisions. Steps to be taken to avoid hernia should include careful closure of the peritoneum and rectus sheath. The avoidance of drainage through the wound where possible, the evacuation of haematomas or abscesses and the prompt use of antibiotics where indicated.

HAEMORRHAGE

The diagnosis of haemorrhage may be immediately apparent if there is revealed bleeding from the abdomen or vagina or it may be suspected by the presence of general cardio-vascular signs such as pallor, restlessness, a feeling of faintness and a rising pulse and falling blood pressure. Primary or immediate post-operative haemorrhage into the abdominal cavity is most likely to be due to a slipped ligature, usually that round the ovarian pedicle while vaginal haemorrhage may be due to bleeding from the lateral vaginal angle after an abdominal hysterectomy or to failure of haemostasis in closing the incision after vaginal repair. Failure to stop bleeding from pedicles at vaginal hysterectomy may require opening of the abdomen. There should be no hesitation in doing this at an early stage in any patient in whom intra-abdominal haemorrhage is suspected. The secondary haemorrhage is caused by septic erosion of some vessel in the operative field. The commonest time for it to occur is around the 10th day and it is more common after vaginal operations such as repair and cone biopsy of the cervix than after abdominal hysterectomy. Secondary haemorrhage may also occur in association with anti-coagulant treatment. This is a particularly unfortunate complication, when anti-coagulants have been given prophylactically in a patient who is thought to be at risk from thrombosis or embolism. There appears to be less danger from the prophylactic use of subcutaneous heparin than from full anti-coagulation with heparin followed by warfarin. Secondary vaginal haemorrhage may be difficult to control with sutures because of the friability of the tissues and packing may then have to be employed.

SEPTIC SHOCK

This has already been discussed in the chapter on infections of the genital tract. The elimination of post-operative sepsis by chemotherapy has helped to reduce the incidence of this serious complication.

THROMBOSIS AND EMBOLISM

Awareness of the dangers of thrombosis and embolism, combined with the practice of genuine, early ambulation, in the post-operative period, has led to the reduction in these dreaded complications. However, it is disturbing that more than half the cases of fatal pulmonary embolism have apparently no previous history of thrombosis and that half of the patients who develop extensive thrombosis have no clinical signs referrable to their lower limbs.

Diagnosis

Chest pain and haemoptysis may give warning of some cases of pulmonary embolism but there are others who die from massive embolism within minutes. This makes it desirable to detect thrombosis in the lower limbs wherever possible. The difficulty of this is that clinical signs may not be apparent. Diagnostic aids include:

1. *Venography* which can show the position and size of a thrombus in the leg veins.
2. *Radio-active fibrinogen.* If a small amount of human fibrinogen labelled with a suitable isotope such as iodine 125 is injected into the peripheral blood it will be concentrated in any thrombus and can be detected by a radiation counter.
3. *Ultrasound.* If a portable ultrasonic fetal heart detector which uses the Doppler effect if placed over blood vessels, the presence of moving blood is indicated by audible sounds. If the transducer is applied over the femoral vein the sudden increase of blood flow produced by pressure on the calf will produce quite a loud noise, if the veins in the calf are patent. This has been used extensively as a screening test for thrombus but is open to the objection that manipulation of the calf may result in the detachment in portions of thrombus.

Prophylaxis of thrombosis and embolism

This starts when the woman is first seen in the outpatient department. Patients at increased risk can often be identified. These include:

1. Women over the age of 40.
2. Women with a previous history of thrombosis or embolism.
3. Fat women.
4. Pregnant women.
5. Women with carcinoma.
6. Women who are taking the contraceptive pill.
7. Women with varicose veins.

Prophylactic treatment with anti-coagulants has varied considerably in recent years. At present the least dangerous and most effective method appears to be the subcutaneous injection of calcium heparin 5000 units, three times a day for seven days, the first injection being given with the pre-medication for the operation. In theatre the use of a head down tilt, careful asepsis, gentleness in handing the tissues and meticulous haemostasis are important factors. Some surgeons and anaesthetists favour the use of an intravenous infusion of Dextran 70 during the operation. Post-operatively, the encouragement of genuine early ambulation, which means active mobilisation and not sitting in a chair at the bedside is the most important measure and the almost universal adoption of this practice has been associated with a reduction in the cases of thrombosis and embolism.

Treatment
The decision to give anti-coagulant treatment for deep vein thrombosis in the immediate post-operative period may be a difficult one, for the treatment carries with it the risk of haemorrhage at the operation site. The safest method to employ is the intravenous infusion of heparin adjusted to give a dose of 1500 units per hour. If bleeding occurs the heparin is immediately stopped and protamine sulphate is given intravenously on the basis of 1 ml of a 1 per cent solution for every 1000 units of heparin. Successful anticoagulation with heparin will prevent formation of further clot. Once anticoagulated, the lower limb can be bandaged to prevent oedema and anti-coagulation can be maintained with warfarin sodium. The initial dose of this drug is 25–20 mg and the maintenance dose varies widely from 3–21 mg as determined by the daily pro-thrombin time or thrombo test. There is some variance of opinion about the duration of treatment which may be continued for six weeks or more.

CARDIAC ARREST

This usually occurs when the patient is still in theatre and demands immediate action. External cardiac massage by direct pressure on the sternum at a rate of 60–70 a minute and ventilation with a 100 per cent oxygen are the immediate measures to be employed. If external cardiac massage fails, internal massage should be performed through the diaphragm if the abdomen is already open or through a separate thoracotomy. In the event of ventricular fibrillation, an external defibrillator is applied to the chest wall. Many general hospitals now have specialised cardiac arrest and shock teams constantly available to deal with acute emergencies. If this kind of help is available, it should be summoned immediately.

RESPIRATORY COMPLICATIONS

Pulmonary embolism has already been mentioned and is really a disease of the circulatory system. Amniotic fluid embolism, if not immediately fatal, may be associated with profuse bleeding. Amniotic fluid escaping into the maternal circulation is thought to cause disseminated intravascular coagulation with thrombosis in the pulmonary vessels. Amniotic embolism may occur during or after labour or at Caesarean section. Treatment tends to be highly specialised. The essential measures are ventilation with oxygen and treatment of the disseminated intravascular coagulation. This may involve sophisticated haematological tests and treatment with heparin, as well as immediate measures, to restore the blood volume.

Pulmonary collapse is a common post-operative complication. Mucus blocks the finer bronchi and the alveolar air is then absorbed with collapse of the segments of lung supplied by the affected bronchi. Secondary infection may then occur. The patient becomes dyspneoic and sometimes cyanosed. She attempts to cough but may be unable to expectorate because of pain. The sound of the bronchial secretions rattling with the chest can be clearly heard. Chest movements are diminished and there is basal dullness and diminished air entry. X-ray will reveal signs of segmental collapse. The main treatment is physiotherapy to encourage the patient to cough while supporting the abdominal wound to reduce pain. Antibiotic treatment may become necessary if the sputum is infected.

Bronchitis and pneumonia are relatively uncommon, as compared to pulmonary collapse and embolism and may be associated with a history of chronic respiratory infection.

GASTRO-INTESTINAL COMPLICATIONS

Vomiting is the most important initial symptom and should never be neglected. It may be caused by the following:

1. *Anaesthesia.* Vomiting due to anaesthesia tends to be immediate and there is a risk of pulmonary aspiration (Mendelson's syndrome) if the patient has not recovered her reflexes.

2. *Peritonitis.* This may become evident two or three days after operation and may be associated with a haematoma wound dehiscence or pelvic cellulitis. Treatment with gastric suction, intravenous drip and antibiotics should be started without delay and any localised abscess should be drained.

3. *Paralytic ileus.* This starts with nausea and vomiting, associated with hyperactivity of the bowel and then with gross distension and absence of bowel sounds. Treatment is conservative with sedation, gastric suction and intravenous fluids and the sooner

these measures are employed the more successful will they be.

4. *Intestinal obstruction.* This causes pain and vomiting of sudden onset. Strangulation of the bowel through some orifice or obstruction by adhesions are the most likely causes. Once the diagnosis is certain, urgent surgical treatment should be carried out.

URINARY COMPLICATIONS

Infection

Post-operative urinary infection is common in gynaecological patients, particularly after repair of prolapse. In these cases, infection is usually secondary to catheterisation which has been necessary to relieve retention of urine. Intermittent catheterisation is associated with a lower incidence of urinary infection than the use of the indwelling catheter. Each time the catheter is passed a specimen of urine should be sent for bacteriological examination.

Retention of urine

This may follow any prolapse repair operation, any vaginal operation which involves packing, any extensive operation for pelvic malignancy which damages the nerve supply of the bladder and also in association with pelvic haematocele or abscess. Some patients have post-operative retention of urine for no organic reason. Retention of urine whatever the cause is a worrying symptom for the patient. Every attempt should be made to reassure that bladder function will return to normal and all patients, other than those who are seriously ill, or who require continuous bladder drainage, should be encouraged to get up and pass urine on a bedside commode or under a shower as soon as possible.

Incontinence of urine

This may be true incontinence due to a fistula or more commonly over-flow incontinence associated with urinary retention. Clinical observation and measurement of residual urine will easily reveal the latter condition.

Anuria

If a patient has not passed urine within 24 hours of operation and if little or no urine is withdrawn on catheterisation, anuria is assumed to be present. This may sometimes be due to shock and hypotension but more commonly occurs in the form of an upper nephron nephrosis as after Caesarean section for pre-eclampsia or abruptio placentae or after septic abortion.

Ureteric Obstruction

This may be difficult to diagnose but if the possibility is suspected, the finding of a hydro-nephrosis on intravenous pyelography or ultrasonic examination of the kidney will be confirmatory.

LATE EFFECTS OF GYNAECOLOGICAL OPERATIONS

These may be physical, related to such features as scarring or retention of foreign bodies, or they may be psychological or a mixture of both. Gynaecological operations have social and psychological effects far beyond their immediate physical effects. Some operations may be followed by specific sexual problems such as dyspareunia after pelvic floor repair and loss of libido after therapeutic abortion. Hysterectomy or sterilisation may produce profound sexual or psychological effects, but these can be reduced by careful selection of cases. Every patient should be given a full, and to her understandable, explanation of the effects of any proposed operation and most patients appreciate such a dialogue with their surgeon. If there is no organic lesion detectable, and yet operation is proposed to relieve symptoms, the patient's agreement must be unreserved. Self-reliant patients are more likely to make a good recovery. Women who are persuaded against their will to have operations, or who expect post-operative problems, are more liable to get them. An important part of gynaecological treatment is post-operative examination by the surgeon who did the operation. This is usually performed about six weeks after the operation and any problems can be discussed at that time. The surgeon's attitude in most cases can be one of cheerful confidence and this is often all that is necessary to complete the cure.

Suggestions for further reading

A series of essays on the 'essentials' of any subject cannot be remarkable for originality and I freely acknowledge my debt to teachers, colleagues and friends. 'I am a part of all that I have met' and plagiarism is sometimes inevitable.

I have found the following books particularly useful and know that they are extensively consulted by students preparing for the MRCOG examination.

Barnes, C. G. (1974) *Medical Disorders in Obstetric Practice*. 4th edition. Oxford: Blackwell.

Dewhurst, C. J. (Ed.) (1976) *Integrated Obstetrics and Gynaecology*. 2nd edition. Oxford: Blackwell.

Donald, I. (1969) *Practical Obstetric Problems*. 4th edition. London: Lloyd-Luke.

Howkins, J. & Stallworthy, J. (1974) *Bonney's Gynaecological Surgery*. 8th edition. London: Ballière Tindall.

Macdonald, R. R. (Ed.) (1978) *Scientific Basis of Obstetrics and Gynaecology*. 2nd edition. Edinburgh: Churchill Livingstone.

Moir, D. D. (1976) *Obstetric Anaesthesia and Analgesia*. London: Ballière Tindall.

Myerscough, P. R. (1977) *Munro Kerr's Operative Obstetrics*. 9th edition. London: Ballière Tindall.

Novak, E. R. & Woodruff, J. D. (Eds.) (1974) *Novak's Gynecologic and Obstetric pathology*. 7th edition. Philadelphia: Saunders.

Novak, E. R., Jones, G. S. & Jones, H. W. (Eds.) (1975) *Novak's Textbook of Gynaecology*. 9th edition. Baltimore: Williams & Wilkins.

Walker, J., MacGillivray, I. & Macnaughton, M. C. (Eds.) (1976) *Combined Textbook of Obstetrics and Gynaecology*. 9th edition. Edinburgh: Churchill Livingstone.

In addition to these standard texts the student will benefit greatly from consulting publications which review rapidly advancing aspects of the speciality. Notable among these are:

Stallworthy, J. & Bourne, G. (Eds.) (1977) *Recent Advances in Obstetrics and Gynaecology*, No. 12. Edinburgh: Churchill Livingstone.

Clinics in Obstetrics and Gynaecology (Specialised subjects under various editors). Published three times yearly. Philadelphia: Saunders.

Obstetrical and Gynaecological Survey. Monthly publication. Baltimore: Williams & Wilkins.

Students should also be aware of current work reported in the major journals such as *The Lancet, The British Medical Journal,*

The British Journal of Obstetrics and Gynaecology, *The American Journal of Obstetrics and Gynecology* and *Obstetrics and Gynecology*. It is good practice to summarise major articles from these journals on postcards.

The proliferation of medical literature is a serious problem of our time. The aspiring specialist must learn to be discriminating in his reading or he will perish from a surfeit of medical jargon. He must be prepared to present a balanced discussion on clinical problems and give his own views clearly and without equivocation.

Index